Experiments and Demonstrations in Physical Therapy

An Inquiry Approach to Learning

STEPHEN E. DiCARLO, P.T., Ph.D.
Wayne State University School of Medicine

REBECCA L. ROSIAN-RAVAS, P.T., M.S.

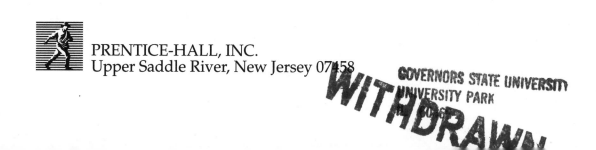

PRENTICE-HALL, INC.
Upper Saddle River, New Jersey 07458

Library of Congress Cataloging-in-Publication Data

DiCarlo, Stephen Edward, 1952–
    Experiments and demonstration in physical therapy : an inquiry
approach to learning / Stephen E. DiCarlo, Rebecca L. Rosian-Ravas.
        p.   cm.
    Includes bibliographical references
    ISBN 0-13-095686-4
    1. Physical therapy—Problems, exercises, etc.   I. Rosian-Ravas,
Rebecca L.   I. Title.
    RM706.D53   1999
    615.8′2—dc21
                                                            98-41442
                                                            CIP

Publisher: *Susan Katz*
Acquisitions Editor: *Mark Cohen*
Editorial Assistant: *Stephanie Camangian*
Marketing Coordinator: *Cindy Frederick*
Marketing Manager: *Tiffany Price*
Director of Production and Manufacturing: *Bruce Johnson*
Managing Production Editor: *Patrick Walsh*
Senior Production Manager: *Janet McGillicuddy*
Creative Director: *Marianne Frasco*
Cover Design: *Miguel Ortiz*
Composition: *BookMasters, Inc.*
Presswork/Binding: *Banta/Harrisonburg*

© 1999 by Prentice-Hall, Inc.
A Simon & Schuster Company
Upper Saddle River, New Jersey 07458

Printed in the United States of America

10 9 8 7 6 5 4 3 2 1

Prentice-Hall International (UK) Limited, *London*
Prentice-Hall of Australia Pty. Limited, *Sydney*
Prentice-Hall Canada Inc., *Toronto*
Prentice-Hall Hispanoamericana, S.A., *Mexico*
Prentice-Hall of India Private Limited, *New Delhi*
Prentice-Hall of Japan, Inc., *Tokyo*
Simon & Schuster Asia Pte. Ltd., *Singapore*
Editora Prentice-Hall do Brasil, Ltda., *Rio de Janeiro*

We wish to extend our sincere appreciation
to Heidi L. Collins, Ph.D., and Ms. Karen
Greene, Department Assistant, in the
Department of Physiology, for their expert
preparation of this manuscript.

Contents

PART I   Introduction

This manual consists of twelve laboratory exercises that integrate research principles, modality application, and therapeutic exercise concepts. The laboratory exercises are designed to complement and supplement existing class lectures and physical therapy laboratories. The laboratory manual is not designed to stand alone. Rather, the specific exercises are designed to reinforce material presented in physical therapy programs by experimentally testing and critically analyzing physical therapy procedures. The idea is to incorporate scientific inquiry and theory into factual learning and application. This method of experimentally testing and critically analyzing procedures to reinforce didactic material is used in many disciplines. For example, most courses in physiology include a laboratory manual to complement and supplement materials learned in the classroom. This physical therapy laboratory manual is similar. However, in addition to reinforcing lecture material, this manual also contains exercises designed to be used in the laboratory component of several physical therapy classes.

The exercises presented utilize experimental and statistical techniques to understand physical therapy modalities and principles of exercise. The individual instructor is encouraged to select specific experiments to reinforce and integrate specific concepts. The experiments may be used as written or the instructor may modify any experiment to suit the unique situation at his or her school. There is no specific order to the presentation of the experiments.

We believe that the experiments presented in this manual can be used as a supplement during the modalities, therapeutic exercise, and research design courses in any physical therapy program. When I was in physical therapy school, we had a large number of laboratories where we learned how to perform physical therapy procedures and apply physical therapy modalities. We would spend an entire laboratory session learning to position the patient (fellow students) and apply hot packs, for example. In contrast, rather than simply learning the mechanics of the procedures, this laboratory manual contains experiments designed to record and analyze the effect of several physical therapy treatments. That is, rather than simply learning how to apply the treatment, the students will also measure the physiological responses and draw conclusions about the procedure. For example, exercises are presented that experimentally test and evaluate physiological responses to therapeutic heat. The students are encouraged to write a report describing their observations. By learning the procedures in this context, students are involved in active learning and will become critical thinkers and consumers of scientific information.

Similarly, the same principles of critically assessing the physiological responses to a treatment may be used in the therapeutic exercise course. In addition to studying the responses of a healthy population, the therapeutic exercise section contains demonstrations and case studies of how special populations respond to exercise. Finally, this manual provides a valuable introduction to a research design course by providing relevant, short-term studies that the students can conduct.

It is important to note that this manual is not designed as a basic instructional tool for modalities, therapeutic exercise, or research components. Rather, this manual is designed to integrate these components into an active learning format. This manual can be used after or during the presentation of the basic instructional components of the individual courses.

Traditional learning is undergoing a transformation in the life science classroom. Physical therapy education is no exception. Physical therapy educators are challenged to design curricula which include a thorough background in physical therapy presented in a manner which contributes to the development of reflective practitioners. The term *reflective practitioner* was introduced by D. Schon in 1987 and used by Jan P. Reynolds in 1993 to describe the ideal physical therapist.[1] The ideal physical therapist is competent in applying physical therapy procedures and is able to apply a scientific knowledge base to analyze patient's needs and solve problems. Students must be taught in a manner that fosters analytical thought processes (formal reasoning). In order for students to develop independent critical thinking skills, educational materials must require the students' active involvement and encourage them to take responsibility for their education. We developed this laboratory manual for physical therapy students with this in mind. The manual was designed to promote critical thinking, enhance problem solving-skills, and strengthen the scientific basis of physical therapy by experimentally testing procedures used by physical therapists.

Schon concluded that educators placed an "overemphasis on technical rationality or the technical knowledge base for professions."[2] Consequently, young professionals are not prepared to handle situations which require more than just technical skills to solve the problem. Schon refers to these situations as "indeterminate zones" of practice. Professional education curricula which are based on technical procedures produce "technical problem solvers" instead of "reflective practitioners." Technical problem solvers are not capable of making decisions in ambiguous health care environments. Although there is no consensus or mandate on the subjects which should be included and those which should be cut, educators share a similar goal of transforming students into reflective practitioners.

An equally important issue in physical therapy education is encouraging physical therapists to continue their education and advance their profession through research. Many therapists have expressed concern over the future of physical therapy due to the lack of research.[3] In order for physical therapy to enter the 21st century as a respected profession, an increased interest in fostering and producing scientific research is necessary. Scientific research will strengthen the theoretical basis for the procedures and treatments used by physical therapists. Members of the task force commissioned by the American Physical Therapy Association on Content of Postbaccalaureate Entry-level Curricula agreed that "information based on sound research should be integrated throughout the curriculum." An interesting and convenient way to incorporate research into the curriculum is to include laboratory experiments based on actual research studies, like the exercises presented in this manual. In this manner, students can perform experiments to discover the scientific basis for the procedures frequently used in physical therapy clinics. Research can be introduced into the curriculum by way of incorporating laboratory experiments which require students to conduct short-term investigations, learn the physiological basis of procedures performed in the clinic, gain experience in employing the correct technique, and develop appropriate professional behaviors through interaction with his or her peers.

While the purpose of this manual is to contribute to the future of physical therapy and the development of reflective practitioners, the approach involves applying physical therapy modalities and procedures and measuring the physiological responses. In this context, students obtain experience in the scientific process, experimental design, physical therapy methods, and data collection and interpretation. The students are also challenged to analyze and assimilate information from figures, answer questions, make calculations, and construct graphs. These exercises engage students in interactive learning and demand a high level of personal investment and responsibility. Finally, these experiments will help support the scientific basis for the procedures and may facilitate research that will directly improve the delivery of health care.

NOTES

1. Schon, *Educating the Reflective Practitioner,* 3–21; Reynolds, "Towards the 21st Century in PT Education," 54–62, 117–118.
2. Schon, *Educating the Reflective Practitioner,* 3–21.
3. Basmajian, "Research of Retrench," 607–10; Hislop, "The Not-So-Impossible Dream," 1069–80; Michels, "Physical Therapy Research," 6.

PART II Educational Approach

This physical therapy laboratory manual is designed to assist student learning using an inquiry-based approach. Inquiry-approach learning places the student in the role of the investigator. The exercises in this manual set the framework, establishing the content area and concepts to be explored. Students ask questions and develop hypotheses, then structure investigations to answer their questions and test their hypotheses. Through inquiry-based activities, students learn how to structure a problem, determine the types of resources needed, carry out investigations, confront ambiguous findings, construct relationships among findings, and create analogies based on their research. Students share their findings with each other, providing opportunities to hone their skills in writing, as well as data manipulation and presentation. Inquiry-approach learning is essential for preparing our students for the 21st century. The explosion of information in recent decades and the promise of continued rapid change in technology and information processing make it imperative that students know how to structure questions, find appropriate information sources, design investigations, analyze findings, and draw conclusions. Learning by inquiry *works*. It has been demonstrated that students who learn by the inquiry approach grasp the basic concepts as well as or better than students who learn by more traditional methods and, as expected, they have better problem-solving skills.[1]

In this context, it is important to point out this physical therapy manual is not designed to cover every or even most components of physical therapy education. It is, however, designed to cover selected topics in depth. Instructors may choose to use this manual for the basis of a graduate level course in physical therapy. Alternatively, instructors may choose to select specific exercises for their modalities, research design, or therapeutic exercise courses. By critically covering a specific topic in depth, students will develop a new philosophy of learning. That is, students will understand that the way a topic is covered is much more important than the actual topic itself. Horace Davenport summed up this concept by stating, "There is a great difference between teaching and learning: there is too much teaching and not enough learning."[2] This represents a fundamental change in America's educational philosophy. Traditional teaching, from kindergarten through professional school, has been described as a mile wide and an inch deep. American textbooks cover 20 to 30 topics and are several hundred pages long. In sharp contrast, similar textbooks in Japan and Germany cover only 5 to 8 topics. Furthermore, American students rely much too heavily on the teacher for their learning. In fact, American students state that the teacher is the single most important factor that determines their ability to learn. Again, in sharp contrast, students in Japan and Germany rely much less on the teacher and state that learning is facilitated by the teacher providing opportunities not dispensing information. This laboratory manual is designed to address these issues. Furthermore, it is hoped that students will no longer function passively, like vessels waiting to be filled with a predetermined body of knowledge. Rather, students must become actively involved in their learning. By becoming actively involved in the learning process, the students enhance their level of understanding and ability to integrate and synthesize material. In addition, the students' conceptualization of function and mechanisms—and ultimately their level of retention—is superior.

NOTES

1. Matjas, "Teaching by Inquiry," 43.
2. Vander, "The Excitement and Challenge of Teaching Physiology: Shaping Ourselves and the Future," S-3–S-16.

PART III Basic Research Design Principles

LABORATORY EXERCISE 1: CORRELATION STUDIES

BACKGROUND AND THEORY

Correlation studies are often conducted to show the relationship between two variables. For example, in this experiment we are going to determine the relationship between the maximum number of sit-ups and the maximum number of push-ups completed by students in this lab. Correlation studies allow us to predict the likelihood of one observation occurring in the presence of the other.

In order to view the degree of relationship between two variables, pairs of values are plotted on a graph. One value of variable X is therefore associated or paired with one value of variable Y. Plotting a number of these points on a graph will generate a scatter diagram (Figure 1-1). If the points resemble a diagonal line, the scatter diagram indicates correlation. Positive correlation is exhibited if Y increases as X increases (Panel A). If Y decreases as X increases, negative correlation exists (Panel B). Zero correlation is shown in the diagram if there is no systematic distribution of the points (Panel C). Therefore, from the scatter diagram we can understand the presence or absence of a relationship between the two observations without performing any calculations. A regression line can be obtained from the scatter diagram by drawing a line of best fit such that there are approximately the same number of points on either side of the straight line. The regression line is useful when only one variable is known. For example, if we knew the value on the X-axis, we could draw a perpendicular line up from that point to the regression line. By drawing a straight line from the point on the regression line to the Y-axis the predicted value of Y can be determined (Figure 1-2).

In order to determine the degree of relationship between the X and Y variables, the **Pearson product-moment correlation coefficient,** r, is often calculated using the following equation,

$$b_0 = \frac{\Sigma y - b\Sigma x}{n}$$

where X is the value of one variable, Y is the value of the second variable, and Σ is the symbol for summation. The r value can be positive or negative, ranging from -1.00 to $+1.00$. If $r = -1$, perfect negative correlation exists. Likewise if $r = +1$, perfect positive correlation exists. Because neither zero nor perfect correlation often exist, we can expect to find some degree of correlation. It is important to remember that the coefficient (r) indicates only the direction of correlation and not the degree;

A.

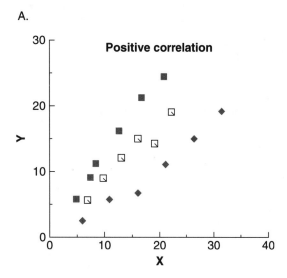

B.

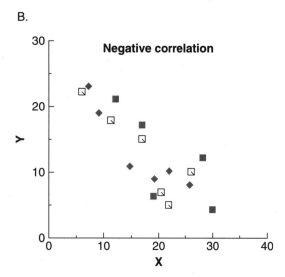

C.

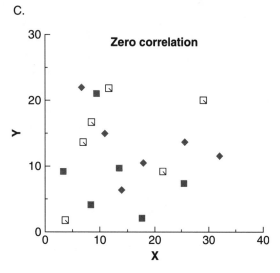

Figure 1-1   Scatter diagrams representing (A) positive, (B) negative, and (C) zero correlation.

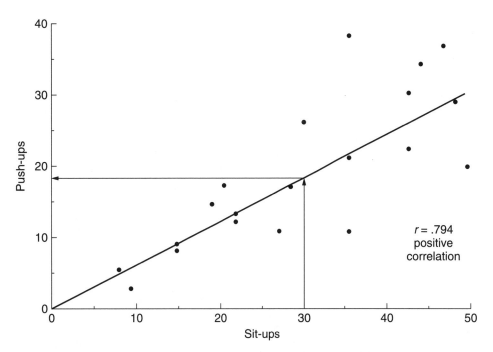

Figure 1-2   Example of a scatter diagram created with one point from student in Group A. Each point represents the number of sit-ups and push-ups completed by one student. If a student in Group B completed 30 sit-ups in thirty seconds, from the graph, we can predict that the student could complete approximately 18 push-ups.

the degree is indicated by the absolute value of r. The coefficient may also be represented by significance levels. For a given sample with degrees of freedom, $df =$ n-2 where $n =$ sample size, a critical value for r can be obtained from a table of critical r values. If the calculated r is greater than the critical r, the correlation is significant, i.e. the relationship between the two variables did not occur by chance.

Materials

gym clothes, mat or towels, stopwatch or timer

Purpose

The purpose of this laboratory experiment is to provide an opportunity to understand and conduct a correlation study. You will benefit from this experiment because you are likely to encounter or devise a correlation study once you begin your clinical work.

Student Objectives

1. To become familiar with correlation studies.
2. To construct a scatter diagram representing the relationship between two variables to determine if the correlation between the variables is positive, negative, or zero.
3. To calculate the correlation coefficient and understand the range that r can be.

4. To use the scatter diagram to predict the likelihood of one variable when the value of a second variable is known.

STEP 1: EXPERIMENTAL PROCEDURES

1. Divide the class into two groups, A and B. Complete Table 1-1 by calculating the mean $\overline{X}$ age, height, and weight for Groups A and B. Also calculate the standard deviation (SD).

   The SD can be calculated using the following equation:

   $$SD = \sqrt{S^2}$$

   $$\text{where, } S^2 = \frac{\Sigma(X_i - \overline{x})^2}{n - 1}$$

   where x_i is the value of one variable, $\overline{x}$ is the mean of the population, n is the sample size, and Σ is the symbol for summation.

2. Students in Group A should pair off and perform the sit-up and push-up exercises described below. Complete Table 1-2 and Figure 1-3. Figure 1-3 will consist of one point from each member of Group A; draw a line of best fit to represent the regression line.

3. The students in Group B should perform only the sit-up exercise and record values on Table 1-3. Using Figure 1-3, predict the number of push-ups that can be achieved based on the number of sit-ups completed. Draw a perpendicular line from the point on the X-axis (which represents the number of sit-ups performed) up to the regression line. Draw another line from the regression line over to the y-axis. This will be the predicted number of push-ups that can be completed based on the number of sit-ups completed. Complete Table 1-3.

4. If time permits, students in Group B can perform the push-up exercise and compare the actual number completed with the predicted number obtained from Figure 1-3.

Sit-up Exercise

1. Lie supine on the mat with knees and hips flexed; feet should be flat on the mat 15–20 cm apart. Your partner should kneel in front of your feet and apply pressure to the instep of each foot to assure that both heels remain on the mat.

Table 1-1 Characteristics of students in Group A and Group B.

	Group A $\overline{X} \pm$ SD	Group B $\overline{X} \pm$ SD
Age (years)		
Height (cm)		
Weight (kg)		
Gender (m/f)		

Table 1-2   Results of sit-up and push-up exercises for students in Group A.

Students in Group A	Maximum number of sit-ups completed	Maximum number of push-ups completed

2. Raise scapulae (shoulder blades) off the mat approximately 14 cm, then return to the starting position.
3. When ready, start the timer and complete as many sit-ups as possible in 30 seconds. Record that value in Table 1-2 (Group A) or Table 1-3 (Group B).

Push-up Exercise

1. Lie prone on the mat and place your hands palm down on the mat beside your shoulders. Push yourself up so that your arms are firmly extended.

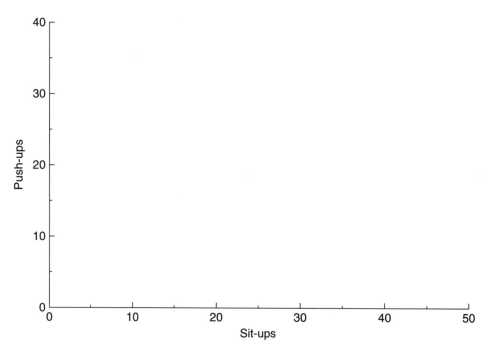

Figure 1-3 Scatter diagram created with one point from each student.

Return to the down position, allowing your chest to touch the mat. Be sure to keep your back, hips, and legs in the same plane throughout the exercise.

(Performing the push-up this way may be difficult for the females in the class; therefore, females may perform the push-up from their knees.)

2. Your partner should place his or her hand beneath your sternum to assure that the down position has been reached; your partner should also check for proper alignment of the legs, hips, and back.

3. When ready, complete as many push-ups as possible in 30 seconds. Record the number completed on Table 1-2.

Constructing the Scatter Diagram

1. Each point will be a pair of values consisting of the maximum number of sit-ups and the maximum number of push-ups. Plot a point on Figure 1-3 for each student in Group A.

2. Determine if the correlation is positive, negative, or zero by calculating r. The calculated r is the observed value and should be compared with the critical value of r in Table 1-4. If the observed r is greater than or equal to the critical r from the table, than the relationship is significant.

3. Predict the number of push-ups each student in Group B can do based on the maximum number of sit-ups completed.

4. Compare the actual number of push-ups with the predicted value.

Table 1-3   Results of sit-up and push-up exercises for students in Group B.

Students in Group B	Maximum number of sit-ups completed	Predicted maximum number of push-ups completed

Table 1-4   Critical values of the Pearson product-moment correlation coefficient. If the observed value of $r \geq$ critical value of r, the correlation is significant, i.e., the relationship did not occur by chance.

| | \multicolumn{5}{c}{Level of significance for two-tailed test} |
$df = n - 2$	.10	.05	.02	.01	.001
1	.9877	.9970	.9995	.9999	1.0000
2	.9000	.9600	.9800	.9900	.9990
3	.8064	.8783	.9343	.9587	.9912
4	.7293	.8114	.8822	.9172	.9741
5	.6694	.7554	.8329	.8745	.9507
6	.6215	.7067	.7887	.8343	.9249
7	.5822	.6664	.7498	.7977	.8982
8	.5494	.6319	.7155	.7646	.8721
9	.5214	.6021	.6851	.7348	.8471
10	.4973	.5760	.6581	.7079	.8233
11	.4762	.5529	.6339	.6835	.8010
12	.4575	.5324	.6120	.6614	.7800
13	.4409	.5139	.5923	.6411	.7603
14	.4259	.4973	.5742	.6226	.7420
15	.4124	.4821	.5577	.6055	.7246
16	.4000	.4683	.5425	.5897	.7004
17	.3887	.4555	.5285	.5751	.6932
18	.3783	.4438	.5155	.5614	.6787
19	.3687	.4329	.5034	.5487	.6652
20	.3598	.4227	.4921	.5368	.6524
25	.3233	.3809	.4451	.4869	.5974
30	.2960	.3494	.4093	.4490	.5541
35	.2746	.3246	.3810	.4182	.5189
40	.2573	.3044	.3578	.3932	.4896
45	.2428	.2875	.3384	.3721	.4648
50	.2306	.2732	.3218	.3541	.4433
60	.2108	.2500	.2948	.3248	.4078
70	.1954	.2319	.2737	.3017	.3799
80	.1829	.2172	.2565	.2830	.3568
90	.1726	.2050	.2422	.2673	.3375
100	.1638	.1946	.2301	.2540	.3211

STEP 2:   *DESIGNING AND CONDUCTING YOUR OWN STUDY*

The following examples may be substituted for the sit-up versus push-up exercise or performed following the completion of the exercise. The following exercise will provide an opportunity for students to perform a correlation study on their own. Students may follow the same steps involved in the sit-up versus push-up correlation example. Be sure students record all measurements in order to construct a scatter diagram and determine the correlation.

1. Correlate height (cm) and vital capacity (ml). With age (during the growth period of an individual), vital capacity increases. As an individual's chest cavity becomes larger, his or her vital capacity increases. Recall that vital capacity is the maximum air that can be expelled following a maximal inspiration. You will need a spirometer to measure the vital capacity.

2. Correlate arm circumference and maximum torque produced during isometric contraction at 60° elbow flexion. The force generated by a muscle is a

function of the size of the individual muscle fibers. You will need an iso-kinetic dynamometer; set the speed at zero in order to measure the torque produced by an isometric contraction.

3. Would the relationships determined in Step 1 be greater if the experiment were conducted in a single sex? The instructor may choose to critically ana-lyze the results obtained from the exercise that determined the relationship between the number of push-ups and sit-ups that an individual could do. The instructor should divide the class into two groups, men and women. After the class is divided into these groups, the original experiment (protocols) should be repeated. The correlation (relationship) between the number of sit-ups and push-ups that an individual can perform should be improved by dividing the groups by sex. The reason for this is that upper body strength, on average, is substantially different between males and females; thus, by separating the groups by sex, the correlation should be improved. Repeating the original exercise in this manner would be an excellent way to introduce the concept of "grouping variables" and their significance and impact on data analysis and outcomes.

4. Design and conduct an experiment. Instructors and students are encouraged to design a correlation study based on relationships that they have observed. This exercise will help students become more actively involved in their education.

⇒ *Point of Interest*

The instructor may also choose to expand the discussion concerning the concepts of "level of significance" and "*p* value."

LABORATORY EXERCISE 2: RELIABILITY OF PHYSICAL THERAPY PROCEDURES

BACKGROUND AND THEORY

The reliability of an experiment must be determined in order for the investigator to confidently interpret his or her results. Reliability refers to the consistency and accuracy of the method of measurement employed in the study. For example, there are numerous studies which discuss the reliability of measuring active and passive joint range of motion (ROM) with the goniometer (Figure 2-1). Although other methods do exist, the universal goniometer is the tool most commonly used by physical therapists to measure range of motion.

Investigators are concerned with the reliability of multiple ROM measurements obtained by a single therapist. This is referred to as **intratester reliability.** In this case, an intraclass correlation coefficient will be calculated to represent the relationship between the multiple measurements; the intraclass correlation coefficient is calculated in the same manner that the correlation coefficient, *r*, was calculated in Laboratory Exercise 1. To better understand intratester reliability, think about the following example. Monday morning a therapist obtains shoulder range of motion measurements on patient A. Tuesday morning the same therapist obtains another set of shoulder ROM measurements on patient A. Are the two sets of measurements the same? By evaluating intratester reliability, we are assessing the consistency and accuracy of the measurements taken by one therapist.

An equally likely situation in the clinic is the possibility of more than one therapist performing ROM measurements on patient A. The therapist working Monday morning obtains shoulder ROM measurements on patient A; however, Tuesday morning a different therapist is working and therefore he or she obtains shoulder ROM measurements on patient A. Assessing the accuracy of the measurements taken by two therapists is referred to as **intertester reliability.** As with intratester reliability, intertester reliability is evaluated by calculating the correlation coefficient, *r*. It is important to remember that although intra- and intertester reliability are determined using the same equation, they are evaluating two different situations.

In the following laboratory exercise, we will test the reliability of measuring shoulder range of motion using the universal goniometer. After each student has learned to correctly use the goniometer, measurements will be performed on each student and reliability will be calculated. Step 2 of this exercise will consist of obtaining reliable chronaxie values. Upon completion of this exercise, each

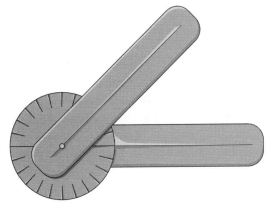

Figure 2-1   Example of goniometer used to measure joint angles.

student should understand and appreciate the importance of obtaining reliable measurements.

Materials

goniometers, calculators, ruler (straight edge)
square wave generator, chronaximeter

Student Objectives

1. To learn how to perform range of motion measurements with the goniometer and obtain consistent measurements.
2. To learn how to obtain chronaxie values and construct strength-duration curves in Step II.
3. To calculate correlation coefficients which assess intratester and intertester reliability.
4. To understand the clinical significance of obtaining reliability.

STEP 1:   EXPERIMENTAL PROCEDURES

The purpose of this laboratory experiment is to provide the student with practical applications of reliability and the opportunity to practice obtaining range of motion measurements and chronaxie/rheobase values.

1. Divide the class into two groups, Group A and Group B.
2. Initially, members of Group A will be the subjects, while students in Group B will be the investigators. The roles will be reversed so that each student has an opportunity to perform the measurements.
3. The subjects should spread out around the room, creating stations through which the investigators can rotate.
4. Members of Group B (investigators) will make two measurements of flexion (see directions below) for each student in Group A. The investigators will rotate through each station taking only one measurement; therefore, two rotations must be completed in order to obtain two measurements.

5. Record values from the first rotation in Table 2-1a. Leave Table 2-1a with your laboratory instructor before proceeding with the second rotation. This will prevent you from being influenced by your first measurements. Record values from the second rotation in Table 2-1b; you do not need to leave this table with your instructor.

6. Students in Group A will then record medial rotation (see directions below) measurements on students in Group B—i.e., reverse roles so that members of Group B are the subjects. The investigators again should rotate through each station twice, recording the first measurement on Table 2-1a and the second measurement on Table 2-1b. Directions to follow when measuring shoulder flexion and medial rotation:

Flexion—0° to 180°

a. The subject should be supine with good postural alignment on the plinth. The subject's palm should face the ceiling while the arm travels anteriorly (Figure 2-2).

b. The student measuring range of motion with the goniometer should place the stationary arm of the goniometer along the midaxillary line of the trunk. Align the axis of the goniometer with the axis of rotation of the shoulder. Rotate the moving arm of the goniometer to lie along the lateral condyle of the humerus, in line with the olecranon process.

Medial Rotation (Internal Rotation)—0° to 90°

a. The subject should be supine on the plinth with shoulder abducted to 90° (Figure 2-3). Flex the elbow to 90° with the palm of the hand facing the body. The forearm should be perpendicular to the table.

Table 2-1a Measurement of joint range of motion for the first rotation.

Student	Range of motion (°)
1	
2	
3	
4	
5	
6	
7	
8	
9	
10	
11	
12	
13	
14	

Table 2-1b   Measurement of joint range of motion for the second rotation.

Student	Range of Motion (°)
1	
2	
3	
4	
5	
6	
7	
8	
9	
10	
11	
12	
13	
14	

Let X = measurements taken from first rotation.
Let Y = measurements taken from second rotation.

b. The student measuring range of motion with the goniometer should place the stationary arm of the goniometer parallel to the support surface. Adjust the goniometer so that the axis is at the olecranon process. Rotate the moving arm of the goniometer so that it lies along the dorsal midline of the forearm between the styloid processes, parallel to the ulna.

Before proceeding with the second rotation, hand Table 2-1a, which you completed earlier, to your laboratory instructor to insure that your second measurements are not influenced by your first measurements.

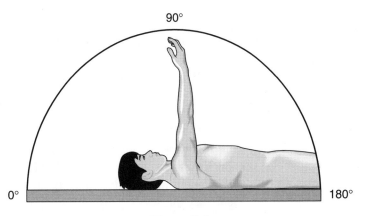

Figure 2-2

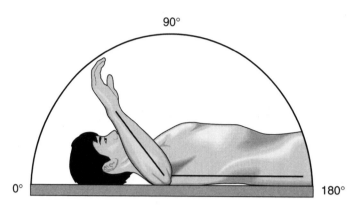

Figure 2-3

Using these measurements, it is possible to calculate the reliability of one student performing the measurement technique. Follow the instructions below to determine intratester reliability, r.

Determining Intratester Reliability

1. Obtain Table 2-1a from your laboratory instructor.
2. You will need the data from Tables 2-1a and 2-1b to complete Table 2-2 and determine intratester reliability.
3. Plot an (X,Y) pair for each student on Figure 2-4. You should recognize from Laboratory Exercise 1 that you are constructing a scatter diagram. Determine if the correlation is positive, negative, or zero.
4. In order to determine intratester reliability, you will calculate the correlation coefficient, r, with the following equation:

$$b_0 = \frac{\Sigma y - b\Sigma x}{n}$$

Let X be the first measurement (from Table 2-1a) and Y be the second measurement (from Table 2-1b). You should have one X and one Y for each student.

5. The coefficient represents intratester reliability, or the consistency of one person obtaining the same measurement of flexion in more than one trial.
6. The correlation coefficient value will fall between zero and one. Zero is the poorest measure of reliability; one is the greatest measure of reliability.

Determining Intertester Reliability

1. Calculating intertester reliability will require members of Group A to pair off and members of Group B to pair off.
2. The pairs should complete Table 2-3 by pooling their first ROM measurements from Table 2-1a. Your first measurement of one subject will be X and your partner's first measurement of the same subject will be Y.
3. Plot an (X,Y) pair for each subject on Figure 2-5 to construct a scatter diagram. Determine if the correlation is positive, negative, or zero.
4. Using the equation shown above, calculate the correlation coefficient, r.

Table 2-2 Let *X* = the first measurement (from Table 2-1a). Let *Y* = the second measurement (from Table 2-1b).

Student	X	Y
1		
2		
3		
4		
5		
6		
7		
8		
9		
10		
11		
12		
13		
14		

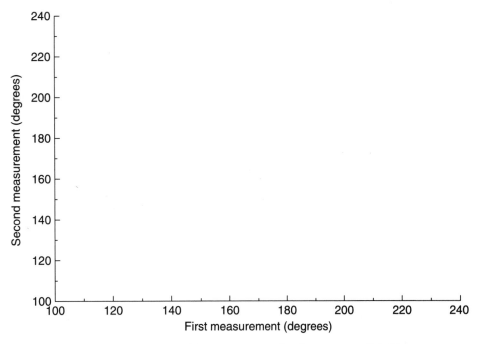

Figure 2-4 Scatter diagram representing intratester reliability.

Table 2-3   Pool the results of measurements taken during the first rotation. Let
X = the measurements obtained by you. Let Y = the measurements obtained by
your partner.

Student	X	Y
1		
2		
3		
4		
5		
6		
7		
8		
9		
10		
11		
12		
13		
14		

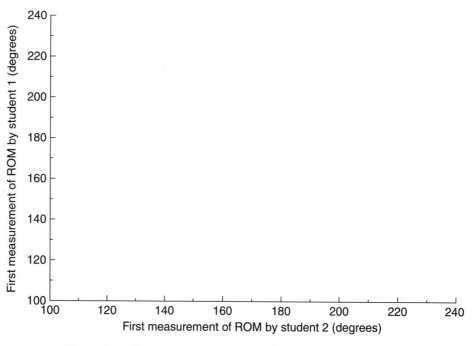

Figure 2-5   Scatter diagram representing intertester reliability.

5. The coefficient represents intertester reliability, or the consistency of results obtained by more than one investigator.

The values on Table 2-3 allow you to calculate the reliability of two students performing the measurement technique. Follow the instructions on page 20 to determine intertester reliability, *r*.

STEP 2:   CHRONAXIE/S-D CURVES

Chronaxie determination with the construction of strength-duration curves allows researchers and clinicians to determine muscle and nerve integrity. Chronaxie determination is based on the concept that the current strength needed to elicit muscle contraction varies inversely with the duration of application of the current. If the current is applied for an infinitely long period of time, the strength of the current can be reduced to a minimum level that will still produce a muscle contraction. **Chronaxie** traditionally is defined as the shortest duration of electrical current required to produce excitation of tissue, when the current strength is twice the rheobase. The **rheobase** refers to the minimal intensity of current of prolonged duration necessary to excite the tissue.

The strength duration curve is a hyperbola which can be constructed knowing only two points, the rheobase and chronaxie. The strength-duration curve can also be created by plotting the strength and corresponding duration of current necessary to obtain a minimal visible contraction. From the strength-duration curve, chronaxie and rheobase can be determined (Figure 2-6).

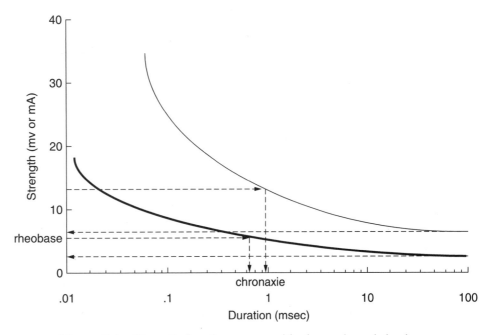

Figure 2-6   Strength-duration curves with chronaxie and rheobase values by arrows. Thick line prepresents the normal condition and the thin line prepresents an impaired neuromuscular condition.

The normal chronaxie value for muscle is .1 msec; values obtained which exceed 1.0 msec are considered to vary significantly from normal. As the excitability of the nerve or muscle is impaired, the chronaxie value increases. An elevation suggests that there is lower motor nerve (alpha motoneuron) damage at some point between the anterior horn cell and the neuromuscular junction, i.e., lead toxicity, Guilain-Barre, or diabetic neuropathy. If there is CNS damage above the lower motor nerve or direct muscle damage, the chronaxie value will not reflect this condition.

The advantages of chronaxie determination are that it is painless for the patient on which it is performed, relatively easy to apply the procedure, and less expensive than EMG equipment. **The major criticism is the difficulty in reproducing the results. Therefore, it would be beneficial to conduct a reliability study on the determination of chronaxie using strength-duration curves. We can determine intratester and intertester reliability as we did with goniometry.**

Subject Preparation

1. Subject should be supine on the plinth with the right leg exposed.
2. Place the dispersive electrode beneath the contralateral gastrocnemius muscle. The dispersive electrode is the inactive electrode which will not be responsible for eliciting the muscle contraction in the right leg. You may see a twitch of the gastrocnemius. Electrode size and stimulus intensity are inversely related to one another. Therefore, if the dispersive electrode is large enough ($>7 \times 12$ cm), the intensity will be minimal.
3. Locate the boundaries of the tibialis anterior muscle by having the subject invert and dorsiflex his or her ankle. The region midway between the distal and proximal muscle attachments will be the region in which the largest contraction can be observed.
4. Stimulate this region at various points to locate the point which produces the greatest contraction with the least amount of current.
5. Shave this region; apply conductive paste and a surface electrode.

Strength-Duration Curve

1. To begin the curve, set current intensity of the generator to zero and pulse width at 300 msec.
2. Gradually increase the current intensity until a minimal visible contraction is seen, i.e., the lowest current that produces a visible contraction. Record the current intensity on Table 2-3a (and 2-3b during the second rotation).
3. Repeat steps 1 and 2 for each pulse width listed in Table 2-3a.
4. Plot the current strength (intensity) required to elicit the minimal visible contraction for each duration on Figure 2-7. Determine rheobase and chronaxie values. Rheobase (mV or mA) will be the intensity of current required to elicit the minimal visible contraction at the pulse width 300 msec. Find the pulse width (duration) on the strength-duration curve which corresponds to the current strength of twice the rheobase. The duration of the pulse is your chronaxie value (msec).

Table 2-3a · Current intensity (mA or mV) for subjects 1–7 from first rotation.

Pulse width (msec)	Subject 1	Subject 2	Subject 3	Subject 4	Subject 5	Subject 6	Subject 7
300							
100							
50							
38							
10							
7							
5							
3							
1							
0.8							
0.6							
0.4							
0.3							
0.1							
0.05							
rheobase							
chronaxie							

Determining Intratester Reliability

1. To determine intratester reliability, the investigator must obtain two chronaxie values and S-D curves from each subject. Therefore, he or she should rotate through the stations set up by each subject. Before rotating through the stations a second time, the investigator must turn in his or her Table 1-3a to the laboratory instructor to prevent bias from the values obtained in the first rotation. The values will be collected on Table 2-3b for the second rotation.

2. Once both rotations have been completed, the investigator can determine intratester reliability (r). Using Tables 2-3a and 2-3b, let X be the chronaxie values obtained during the first rotation and Y be the chronaxie values obtained during the second rotation.

Determining Intertester Reliability

1. Pair up with another investigator; transfer both of your results from the first rotations (values from Table 2-3a) to Table 2-4 on page 30.

2. Calculate intertester reliability (r). Let X be the chronaxie values you obtained from the first rotation and Y be your partner's chronaxie values from the first rotation.

Table 2-3b Current intensity (mA or mV) for subjects 1–7 from first rotation.

Pulse width (msec)	Subject 1	Subject 2	Subject 3	Subject 4	Subject 5	Subject 6	Subject 7
300							
100							
50							
38							
10							
7							
5							
3							
1							
0.8							
0.6							
0.4							
0.3							
0.1							
0.05							
rheobase							
chronaxie							

Let X = chronaxie values for subjects 1–7 obtained in the first rotation (values from Table 2-3a).

Let Y = chronaxie values for subjects 1–7 obtained in the second rotation.

STEP 3: DESIGNING AND CONDUCTING YOUR OWN STUDY

The instructor and students are encouraged to design a study which determines the reliability of other physical therapy procedures. How reliable are the muscle testing procedures? How reliable are gait, posture, or balance evaluation procedures? How reliable is the determination of the 10 repetition maximum or isokinetic units? To conduct these reliability studies, students should review and practice the specific procedure of interest (gait or posture evaluation etc.), then follow the instructions for conducting reliability studies in Steps 1 and 2.

The instructor may choose to compare the reliability of measuring ROM from a different joint with the reliability of measuring ROM from the shoulder (all other procedures would be identical). Technically, measuring internal and external rotation of the shoulder joint is difficult due to the complexity of the shoulder and the difficulty in stabilizing the shoulder to prevent substitutions. Due to the difficulty of measuring ROM from the shoulder, we predict that measures of reliability will be greater when recording ROM from other joints. Test it and find out!

Finally, the instructor may choose to point out the limitations in the procedure of having students rotate from test station to test station and doing the same test in the same sequence. These procedures violate a basic tenant of statistical analysis called "random sampling." The instructor may choose to avoid this limitation by having random station and testing assignments (although this may become very confusing). If this is done, the instructor can compare results obtained without random sampling with the identical procedure using random sampling. In this way, the instructor would introduce and test the concept of order effects and random samples.

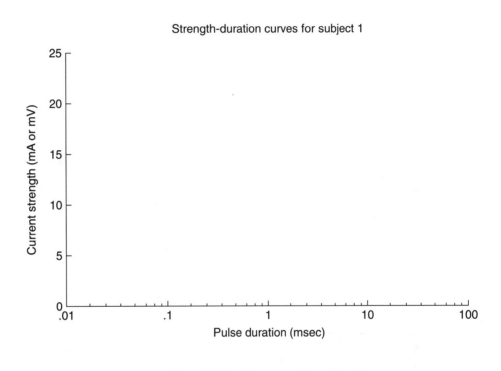

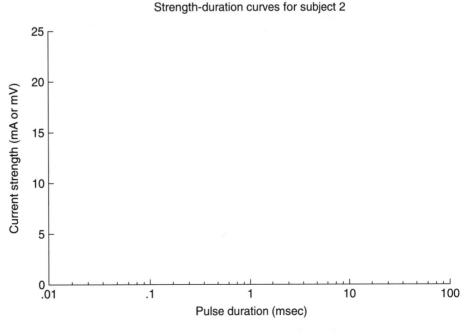

Figure 2-7   Strength-duration curves for subjects 1–7.

Strength-duration curves for subject 3

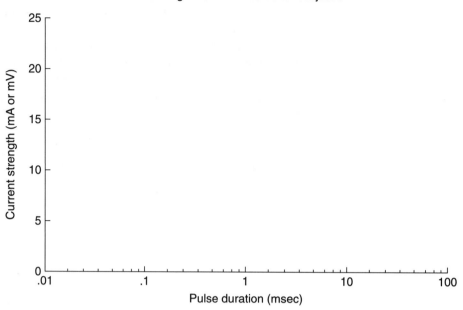

Strength-duration curves for subject 4

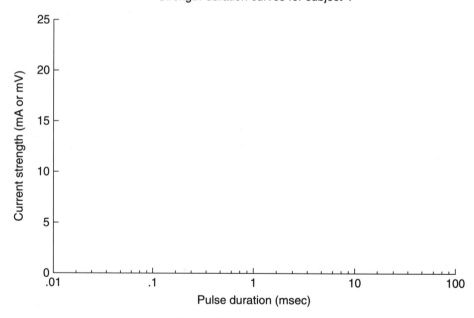

Figure 2-7   continued

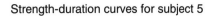

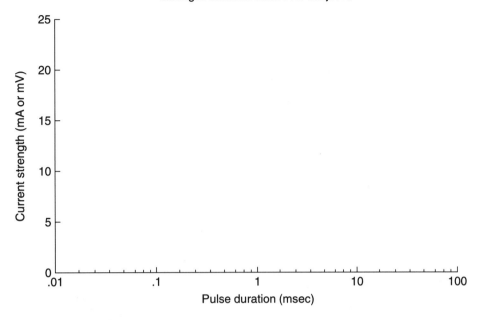

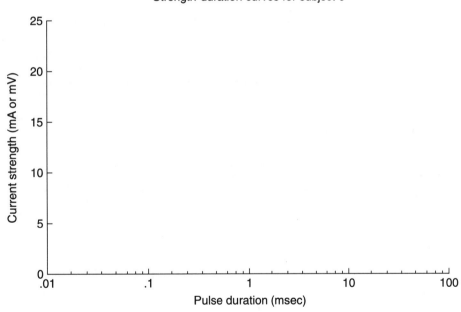

Figure 2-7   continued

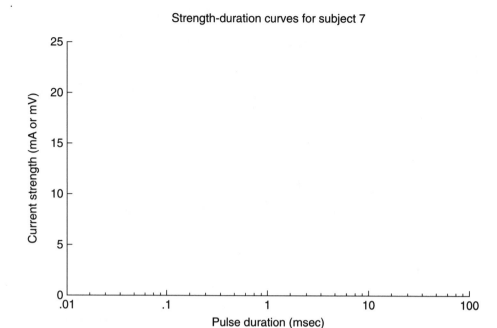

Figure 2-7   continued

Table 2-4   Pooled data (yours and your partner's) from the first rotation.

Student	Investigator's chronaxie value (msec) X	Partner's chronaxie value (msec) Y

Let X = chronaxie values obtained by the investigator in the first rotation.
Let Y = chronaxie values obtained by your partner in the first rotation.

⇒ *Point of Interest*

Pearson product-moment correlation (r) is a simple correlation coefficient that is often used to determine reliability. However, the preferred and accepted method for assessing intra- or intertester reliability is the "Intra- or Interclass Coefficient (*ICC*)." The *ICC* assesses and parcels out variability with respect to true measures versus error. Although the simple correlation has no ability to do this, the simple correlation is an educationally sound way to teach methods for assessing relationships between two variables. However, the instructor may choose to point out the difference between r and *ICC*.

LABORATORY EXERCISE 3:   SINGLE CASE STUDIES

BACKGROUND AND THEORY

Although there are many possible experimental designs, the single case design is commonly used by physical therapists for clinical research. The single case study is an intensive study of one individual to determine if a prescribed treatment is effective. The single case study may be conducted utilizing the A–B–A design, a research design divided into three consecutive time periods, Figure 3-1. The first period, "A," is the baseline period; during this time, the behavior or response will be recorded without treatment intervention to establish a stable or baseline condition. The second period, "B," is the time span over which the treatment is given and the response is continuously monitored. The results can be plotted daily on a graph, where time is the independent variable (X) and the measured response is the dependent variable (Y). The goal of the therapist is to determine whether the intervention had a significant effect on the measured variable, i.e., greater range of motion. The final segment—"A," of the A–B–A design—consists of withdrawal of the intervention. If the intervention had a significant therapeutic effect, then removal of the intervention should result in the measured variable returning back to baseline. The baseline measurements may not be obtained in the third period if the response was learned or the affliction cured. The A–B–A design assumes that the behavior or response being measured is reversible and that all other factors have been addressed, i.e., emotional state or natural improvement in health.

Classical experimental designs require experimental and control groups for comparison testing, and large sample sizes to assure reliability. The difficulty of obtaining large samples of patients with similar conditions (age, sex, medical history) in the clinical environment limits the use of classical experimental designs. The clinical environment lends itself to single case studies because the goal of the therapist is to treat his or her patient effectively. Even if large sampling populations were available in the clinic to study the effectiveness of a given treatment, it is difficult to justify withholding that treatment to a group of patients in order to have a control group for statistical comparison. The disadvantage of the single case design is the difficulty in performing comparison studies. Case studies of patients with the same criteria (age, medical history . . .) can be compared; however, the statistics used in performing these comparison tests are more involved than we will learn at this time.

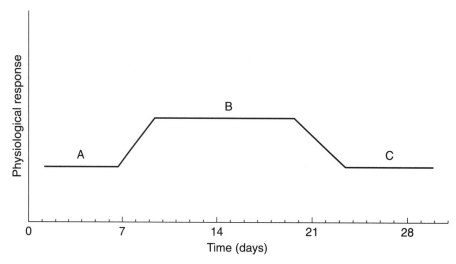

Figure 3-1   Predicted results of an A–B–A design.

The laboratory exercise will be performed over a period of four weeks. We will study flexibility in response to a simple exercise sequence (treatment). The A–B–A design will be the basis to determine if daily exercise is effective in improving flexibility.

Materials

meterstick, tape
EMG recording equipment, electrodes

Student Objectives

1. To learn how to perform clinical research with the single case study.
2. To utilize the A–B–A design to determine the effectiveness of a treatment.
3. To complete a single case study to determine if flexibility can be enhanced with an exercise program consisting of three basic stretches.

STEP 1:   EXPERIMENTAL PROCEDURES

The purpose of this laboratory experiment is for each student to be involved in a single case study as the subject and researcher, and apply the A–B–A design to his or her experiment. **An explanation of the flexibility test and exercise program follows. Please read the directions carefully before proceeding with the experimental procedure.**

Flexibility Test and Exercise Program

1. *DAYS 1–7.* Measure flexibility with the sit and reach test every day for seven days. Record values on Table 3-1, and plot the results on Figure 3-2. This is the baseline or "A" period of the research design.
2. *DAYS 8–21.* Begin doing the stretching exercise program daily and perform the sit and reach test daily. Record values on Table 3-1 and plot the results on Figure 3-2. We will see if daily exercise increases flexibility during this time, period "B."

Table 3-1 Daily flexibility measurements.

Day	Flexibility (cm)	Day	Flexibility (cm)
1		15	
2		16	
3		17	
4		18	
5		19	
6		20	
7		21	
8		22	
9		23	
10		24	
11		25	
12		26	
13		27	
14		28	

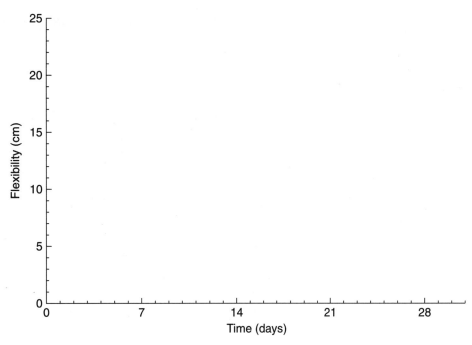

Figure 3-2 Plot of daily flexibility measurements for three periods, A–B–A.

3. *DAYS 22–28.* Discontinue the daily exercise program, but perform the sit and reach test daily. Record flexibility measurements on Table 3-1 and plot the results on Figure 3-2. The results may return towards baseline. This demonstrates that the exercise was effective in increasing flexibility; this is the final period, "A."

Flexibility Test (Sit and Reach)

Total body flexibility is difficult to measure because flexibility is joint specific. However, the Trunk Forward Flexion Test has been modified throughout the years since its introduction in 1941 by Curet. The most recent flexibility test is described below.

1. Place a meterstick on the floor. To secure the meterstick on the floor, place tape at right angles at the 35 cm mark. Participant should warm up with stretching exercises to prevent muscle pulls and back strain.
2. The participant should remove his or her shoes and socks and sit on the floor with legs extended.
3. The participant should sit with the yardstick between the legs so that the 0 mark is toward his or her body. Feet should be 30 cm apart and the participants heels should nearly touch the taped line at the 3 cm mark.
4. With one hand overlapping the other to prevent trunk rotation, the participant should slowly reach forward, touch the meterstick with his or her fingertips, and hold for 2 seconds. The most effective stretch will be performed when the participant exhales and drops his or her head while reaching. Another individual is needed during the test to hold down the participants knees to insure that the knees remain extended.
5. The score is the farthest point reached with the fingertips. The best of three trials is recorded.

Exercise Program

1. *HAMSTRING STRETCH*–to stretch the muscles in the posterior thigh.
   a. The most effective hamstring stretches involve the elimination of gravity. If you are performing a hamstring stretch while standing, the muscle is already partially active or shortened. It is difficult to stretch a muscle which is already shortened. Find a flat surface to sit on such that the edge of the surface is directly behind the flexed knee.
   b. Lean over, touching your chest to your thighs. Extend one leg as far as possible; you should feel the stretch in the back of the leg; hold for 10 seconds.
   c. With the leg still extended slowly raise your upper body about 6 cm. This will release the stretch on the hamstring; you will be able to further extend your knee and stretch your hamstring at another point. Hold for 10 seconds.
   d. During the exercise you are gaining a maximal hamstrings stretch utilizing the reciprocal inhibition characteristics of muscle groups. Contraction of an agonist muscle is associated with inhibition of the antagonist muscle. Notice that as you extend your leg, the muscles of your thigh (quadriceps) contract and the muscles in the posterior leg, i.e., hamstrings are inhibited; this assures that we are effectively stretching the relaxed hamstring.
   e. Repeat the exercise with each leg 5 times, alternating legs.

    2. *KNEE TO CHEST RAISE*–to stretch back muscles.
      a. Lie supine with knees and hips flexed. Feet should be flat on the floor, 30 cm apart.
      b. With both hands pull right knee to chest; hold for count of 5 seconds, then slowly lower to starting position; repeat 5 times.
      c. With both hands, pull left knee to chest; hold for count of 5 seconds, then slowly lower to starting position; repeat 5 times.
      d. With hands on knees pull both knees to chest; hold for 5 seconds, then slowly lower to starting position; repeat 5 times.
    3. *HAMSTRING STRETCH II*–to stretch the muscles of the posterior leg.
      a. Sit on floor with legs extended; arms can be extended parallel to legs or raised alongside the head.
      b. Bend from the waist; attempt to touch your nose to your knees. Knees should be extended; hold this position for 10 seconds.
      c. Slowly raise your body up to the starting position. Repeat procedure 10 times.

Results

In order to analyze the results among students, more sophisticated statistical procedures may be performed which we will not discuss at this time. However, Figure 3-2 can be used to assess the effectiveness of exercise on flexibility, based on the curve generated from the daily measurements. You will be able to determine whether the exercise program altered your own flexibility. Ideally you would see a baseline curve during period A with minor fluctuations. With exercise, the curve generated in the B period should be rising or shifted upward. Removal of the exercises should generate a curve in the third period which resembles the baseline. The conclusion would be that exercise is an effective method of increasing flexibility.

Exercise Test and Training Program

As an alternative to the flexibility test, a strength training program can be performed. The measured variable will be the electrical activity elicited during an isometric contraction. The intervention period will consist of introducing a strength training program (progressive resistance exercises). This study will last six weeks, one week for the baseline period (A), three weeks for the intervention period (B), and two weeks for the return to baseline (A) following the removal of the intervention.

    Numerous studies have been conducted to determine the immediate and prolonged effects of muscle strength training on EMG activity and muscle hypertrophy. It is well established that muscle hypertrophy occurs as a result of strength training; therefore, it is tempting to assume that an increase in muscular strength is due to muscle hypertrophy. However, within the first several weeks of a training program, the increase in force development has not been shown to be associated with an increase in muscle mass. This suggests that the increased strength is due to other muscular or neuromuscular adaptations. Previous studies have indicated that the number of fibers recruited increases and possibly produces a more synchronous firing of motor units with strength training. Early changes

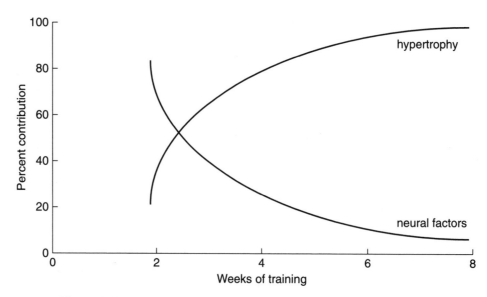

Figure 3-3   Relative contribution of neural and hypertrophic factors during the time course of training.

in strength gain are largely due to neural factors, while the contribution of the hypertrophic factor gradually increases with continued training. Figure 3-3 depicts the relative contributions of neural and hypertrophic factors during the time course of training.[1]

An interesting phenomenon occurring as a result of resistance training is contralateral or cross education of the muscle in the opposite arm being trained. This concept will be demonstrated in the six week study. EMG activity will be recorded in the biceps not being trained. Many researchers have observed an increase in EMG activity in the contralateral limb without an increase in muscle mass. Some results suggest that this phenomenon is due to neural factors which result in higher muscle activation.[2]

Exercise Test

1. *DAYS 1–7.* Measure the integrated EMG (IEMG) activity during maximal isometric contraction at 0° in the right and left biceps every day for seven days. Record values on Table 3-2, and plot the results on Figure 3-4. This is the baseline or "A" period of the research design.

2. *DAYS 8–28.* Perform the progressive resistance exercise (PRE) program daily; measure the integrated EMG activity during maximal isometric contraction at 0° in both arms each day. Record values on Table 3-2 and plot them on Figure 3-4. We will see if strength training increases EMG activity during this time, period "B."

3. *DAYS 28–42.* Discontinue the daily exercise program, but record the peak EMG activity during maximal isometric contraction at 0° for the right and left biceps daily on Table 3-2 and plot them on Figure 3-4. If baseline is achieved then the exercise was effective in increasing EMG activity, i.e. recruitment of more motor units; this is the final period, "A."

Table 3-2 EMG activity (mV) for right and left biceps during six weeks.

Day	Right	Left	Day	Right	Left
1			22		
2			23		
3			24		
4			25		
5			26		
6			27		
7			28		
8			29		
9			30		
10			31		
11			32		
12			33		
13			34		
14			35		
15			36		
16			37		
17			38		
18			39		
19			40		
20			41		
21			42		

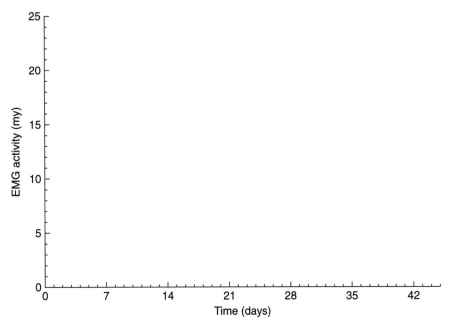

Figure 3-4 Plot of daily EMG values for three periods, A–B–A.

Training Program (Progressive Resistance Exercise Program)

Determine the 10 repetition maximum (10 RM) for right elbow flexors during a biceps curl. The progressive resistance exercise (PRE) program consists of completing three sets of 10 repetitions of increasing loads. The first set of repetitions will be performed at 50% of the 10 RM. The second set of repetitions will be performed at 75% of the 10 RM and the final set will be the 10 RM. Perform the PRE for elbow flexors twice a day, three days per week. Only the right arm should participate in the PRE. After two weeks, retest your maximum strength. If the 10 RM has changed, then adjust the training work load to maintain the 50%, 75%, and 100% maximal load.

STEP 2: DESIGNING AND CONDUCTING YOUR OWN STUDY

The instructor and students are encouraged to design and conduct a study using the A–B–A design or other design learned in their classes.

⇒ Point of Interest

It is important to point out to the students that single case studies are NOT the only experimental designs used by the therapists in research. Students should also know that many other experimental designs are available for and used by physical therapists doing clinical research.

It should also be pointed out that from a clinical prospective, an A–B–A design is often unlikely inasmuch as treatment strategies (i.e., the intervention variable) are likely to be continued.

Finally, it should be pointed out that the use of peak EMG amplitude is a crude and possibly suspect index of performance. A more appropriate measure is integrated EMG. The instructor may choose to discuss the merit of these measurements.

Explanation of the Cross-Transfer Theory

There is a theory of cross-transfer which states that muscles which are not being exercised also increase in strength. This theory refers specifically to the analogous muscles on the opposite side of the body to those muscles being exercised. In other words, if the right arm is trained, the left arm will also increase in strength. Why?

Muscles increase in strength through two processes. The first is probably the most well known. Muscle fibers will enlarge with repeated use; this is **hypertrophy.** There is no increase in the number of fibers so the size increase is due to the muscle fibers becoming larger. For a muscle to increase in strength, it must lift a load; that is why weight lifters have large, well-defined muscles.

However, there is an increase in strength that occurs before there is a noticeable increase in muscle size. This occurs because of changes in the nervous system. Usually the nervous system can only recruit a percentage of the muscle fibers for the action that it wants to perform. With an increased load on the muscle, the nervous system is able to recruit a larger percentage of the available fibers. Recruitment of more fibers increases the strength of the muscle.

As the theory states, there is a strength increase in the unexercised muscle. It seems that the nervous system is able to recruit more fibers in both limbs. The body is always trying to maintain a steady-state or remain balanced. In this case, the nervous system sends action potentials to both arms. However, some people do not have the same build on each side of their bodies. For instance, a pitcher has a larger pitching arm. Initially both arms gained in ability to recruit fibers; however, the exercised arm continued to increase in size (hypertrophy).

NOTES

1. As determined by Moritani and DeVries; see "Neural Factors Versus Hypertrophy," 115–30.
2. Moritani and DeVries, "Neural Factors Versus Hypertrophy," 115–30.

PART IV Clinical Applications: Modalities

LABORATORY EXERCISE 4: PHYSIOLOGICAL RESPONSES TO THERAPEUTIC HEAT

BACKGROUND AND THEORY

As a physical therapist, you will be concerned with minimizing the pain/discomfort that a patient is experiencing. A major mechanism for pain relief is the absorption of energy with subsequent effects. One idea is to add sufficient energy to the patient, providing an increase in nonpainful sensory input to override the painful sensory input. Agents such as heat, water, ultrasonic energy, nerve, and muscle stimulating currents function by this mechanism. This exercise will concentrate only on the application of heat as a therapeutic agent. You may already be familiar with the use of hot packs, the paraffin bath, the whirlpool, and infrared lamps as sources of heat; the thermal energy generated by these sources is transmitted to the patient with the intention of producing a beneficial reaction through cutaneous nervous and circulatory stimulation. Absorption of these forms of thermal energy results in muscle relaxation and therefore pain relief in situations of muscle spasm. However, the depth of penetration by any of these forms is limited to 1 cm. Therefore, muscle relaxation is not the result of direct absorption of energy by the muscle, but due to the direct effect of heat on the cutaneous nerve receptors and blood vessels.

The application of heat produces vasodilation by two mechanisms. Heat acts as an irritant stimulating the dermal mast cells to release a histamine-like substance which causes local dilation. The exposed area will redden. The reddening is referred to as **hyperemia.** The local response is due to a tissue temperature rise at the site of heat application. With prolonged heating over a broad area, the warmed blood will reach the thermoregulatory centers in the hypothalamus. The warmed blood signals an increase in temperature and as a result vasodilation occurs in deeper tissues beneath the exposed area providing increased blood flow to the tissue and systemic **vasodilation** as a means to dissipate heat. Warmth receptors located beneath the skin are stimulated at temperatures above 30°C. Receptor stimulation is believed to be a result of alterations in cell metabolic rate brought about by the temperature change. A 10°C change in temperature alters the rate of intracellular chemical reactions more than twofold. When a large area is exposed to a temperature change, the thermal signals from the entire area summate; this is the concept of **spatial summation of thermal sensations.** Therefore, a temperature change as little as .01°C can be detected if it affects a large area. Nerve conduction velocity may increase in response to a temperature change; however, the receptor also has the capacity to adapt to steady state temperature. Within seconds the strong stimulation of the warmth receptors by heat fades and there is diminished nerve activity.

Hyperemia is not the only visual change which could occur as a result of applying heat to a region. A warning signal to discontinue heat application is the presence of a network of white and red blotches in the exposed area, referred to as **mottling.** The mechanism underlying mottling is rebound vasoconstriction; it is a result of the vessel being maximally dilated for a prolonged period (over thirty minutes). More specifically, the maximally dilated vessel will go into spasm which leads to vasoconstriction and closing of the associated capillaries.

When considering the different modalities available for treatment, generally, the longer the wavelength emitted from a source, the greater the penetration. Wavelength is inversely proportional to frequency, $\lambda = v/f$ where λ is wavelength, v is velocity, and f is frequency. The frequency with which molecules vibrate is proportional to the temperature at that time, i.e., as temperature increases, frequency increases. With these two relationships, the relationship between wavelength and temperature is evident. Wavelength is inversely proportional to the temperature. For example, compare the energy emitted from a cold pack with the energy emitted from a hot pack. The frequency of the waves emitted from the hot pack is greater than the frequency of the waves emitted from the cold pack.

Which modality, the hot pack or the cold pack, penetrates more deeply?

The cold pack penetrates deeper than the hot pack because the cold pack emits energy of longer wavelength than the hot pack.

In this exercise we will examine **luminous** and **non-luminous** heating sources which emit wavelengths in the infrared region of the electromagnetic spectrum (Figure 4-1). Other heat modalities also emit energy within the infrared region. Table 4-1 lists the type of heat modality with its corresponding wavelength, frequency, temperature, and relative depth of penetration. Radiant energy within the IR region will be absorbed up to 95% by the skin; less than 5% is transmitted and reflected. Before proceeding with the experiment, be certain that you understand the relationships among wavelength, temperature, frequency, and depth of penetration.

An exception to the rule that the longer the wavelength, the greater the depth of penetration, exists with the use of luminous and non-luminous heat lamps. The luminous source refers to a high temperature generator that emits shorter wavelengths which fall in the near infrared (IR) region (NIR 770–1,400 nm, 10^{-9}). The non-luminous source requires 10–15 minutes to reach its maximum temperature and emits longer wavelengths which fall in the far infrared region (FIR 1,400–40,000 nm, 10^{-9}). The rule states that the longer the wavelength, the greater the penetration of that energy; this implies that FIR due to its longer wavelength would penetrate to a greater extent than near infrared. However, due to certain unique characteristics of human skin, infrared at a wavelength of 1,200 nm penetrates at a depth greater than longer or shorter wavelengths. Note: This is the *exception* to the rule! For the same intensity of radiant heating, emissions of the far IR may feel warmer than near IR emissions because of greater warming of the superficial nerve endings.

As a therapeutic device to relieve muscle spasm, heat ultimately causes muscle relaxation. The increased blood flow, as a result of local heating, facilitates clearance of metabolites and oxygen delivery to the tissue. The addition of heat has been

Wavelength (λ)
(nm 10^{-9})

Infrared	Far infrared	1,500 – 12,000
	Near infrared	770 – 1,500
Visible light		390 – 770
Ultraviolet light		180 – 390
X-rays	Diagnostic X-ray	0.3 – 1.2
	Therapeutic X-ray	0.5 – 1.5
Gamma rays		0.1 – 0.2

Figure 4-1 Portion of electromagnetic spectrum illustrating the wavelength of different forms of energy.

shown to reduce pain, decrease stiffness of the joints, and increase extensibility of the tendons. Its use in the clinic is vast, from alleviating the pain of patients with muscle strains, fractures, and arthritis, to its essential use prior to massage, voluntary exercise, and passive muscle exercise.

Materials

luminous (near infrared or NIR) heat source
non-luminous (far infrared or FIR) heat source
towels, skin thermometers, timers

Table 4-1 Modalities which emit energy in the infrared region of the electromagnetic spectrum are listed below with their corresponding temperature (T), frequency (f), wavelength (λ), and relative depth of penetration.

Modality	T (°C)	f (m/sec)	λ (nm)	Relative depth of penetration
Cold pack	7.0	2.9×10^{13}	10,307	+ + + +
Paraffin bath	47	3.32×10^{13}	9,019	+ + +
	57	3.43×10^{13}	8,745	+ + +
Hot pack	67	3.53×10^{13}	8,488	+ +
Far infrared	727	1.05×10^{14}	2,860	+ +
Near infrared*	1,727	3.12×10^{14}	962	+ + +

* Near infrared is an exception to the rule. Even though near infrared emits shorter wavelengths, the energy penetrates greater than energy emitted from a far infrared source.

Student Objectives

1. To become familiar with infrared heating as a tool used by the physical therapist.
2. To understand the physiological effects of heat application.
3. To compare NIR and FIR heating.

STEP 1: EXPERIMENTAL PROCEDURES

The purpose of this laboratory exercise is to demonstrate the different responses to two methods of superficial heating.

1. Subject should be prone with both feet off the edge of the plinth; right and left calves should be exposed. To prevent lumbar lordosis, a pillow may be placed beneath the abdomen.
2. The luminous lamp will be used on the right calf; the non-luminous lamp will be used on the left calf.
3. Position both lamps according to the Cosine and Inverse Square Laws.

   Cosine Law—For optimum radiation, the heat source needs to be positioned at a right angle to the surface of the calves.

   Inverse Square Law—The intensity of radiation varies inversely with the square of the distance from the source. Doubling the distance between the source of radiant energy and the patient results in quadrupling the area covered, whereby the intensity drops by 1/4 per unit area. Record the intensity and area of each source. Adjust the heights of the lamps such that the square of the distance between the source and the subject divided into the output wattage is equal. Wattage refers to the power emitted from the lamp. The wattage may be written on the lamp or the wattage can be calculated by multiplying the amperage and voltage together ($W = v * A$). The amperage should be written on the lamp.

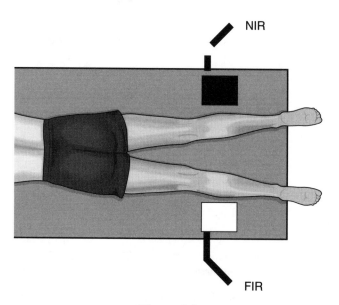

Figure 4-2

Table 4-2 Results of 20 minute heat exposure.

Time (min)	Left calf (°)	Right calf (°)	Observations/ subject's reaction
Initial (no heat)			
5			
10			
15			
20			

4. Drape a towel on the NIR source to prevent airflow across the exposed area and cross contamination from the two lamps.

5. Record the surface temperature of right and left calves prior to heat application. Record in Table 4-2.

6. Turn on both lamps; set timer for 20 minutes.

7. Every 5 minutes, record the temperature of both calves on Table 4-2. Also record any physical changes in the exposed area and how the subject perceives the heat (Table 4-2).

8. At the end of 20 minutes, turn off and unplug the lamps.

9. Construct a bar graph representing the maximum temperature change obtained with NIR and FIR heat sources in Figure 4-3.

General Considerations

1. Do not allow the distance between the heat source and the subject to be less than 50 cm.

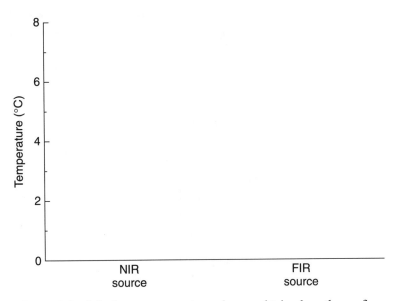

Figure 4-3 Maximum temperature change obtained on the surface of legs using near and far infrared heat sources.

2. Carefully observe the calf for breaks in the skin or scars. Areas of scarring may be more sensitive to the heat.

3. If mottling occurs, place a towel over the calf to decrease the temperature.

4. Remember that the FIR source requires 10 minutes to reach its maximum temperature.

Questions

1. Describe the temperature change which occurred on each calf.

2. Was the temperature change in the left calf different from that in the right calf?

3. If there was a difference, explain the effect in terms of applying heat from an NIR and an FIR source.

4. Did mottling occur?

5. How did the subject perceive the temperature change? Was there a difference between the right and left calves?

6. Explain, physiologically, what occurs as the temperature changes.

$\Longrightarrow$ *Point of Interest*

Although luminous and non-luminous lamps are rarely used as heating modalities, the discussion and procedures provide solid physical principals concerning all thermal modalities. Furthermore, the procedures foster active learning, small-group discussion, and interaction with experimental design, data collection, and analysis.

STEP 2:   THE EFFECTS OF DIRECT AND INDIRECT HEAT ON BLOOD FLOW

This exercise is designed to examine the effect of indirect and direct heat on blood flow. This will be achieved by immersing the student's right hand in warm water and recording the temperature in the left hand. The left hand will be exposed during the first experiment in which indirect heating of the left hand should occur. The left hand will be covered during the second experiment.

1. Fill a bucket or small pail about one-third full of warm tap water at a temperature between 42° and 45°C. Use an alcohol thermometer to monitor the temperature.

2. Using a surface thermometer, record the initial skin surface temperature of the back of the left hand. Record this in Table 4-3.

3. The student should place his or her right hand in the bucket of water. Keep the hand in the bucket for the next 20 minutes. Maintain the 42°–45°C temperature by adding more warm water as needed.

4. Record temperature readings on the left hand once each minute for the next 20 minutes.

Table 4-3   Temperature change in the bare and covered left hand.

Time (min)	Left hand (bare)	Left hand (covered)
0		
1		
2		
3		
4		
5		
6		
7		
8		
9		
10		
11		
12		
13		
14		
15		
16		
17		
18		
19		
20		

5. After 20 minutes, the student should remove his or her right hand from the water and allow time for both hands to return to their initial temperatures.

6. Repeat the above activity, but this time cover the left hand with a towel or blanket. For best results, make sure the legs and arms are also covered (long pants, sweatshirt).

7. Record temperature readings on the left hand each minute for the next 20 minutes. Uncover only a small portion of the left hand when taking the temperature.

8. Using the data from Table 4-3 obtained from the measurements of the bare and covered left hand, make two line graphs on Figure 4-4. Use a solid line to represent the bare hand and a dashed line to represent the covered hand.

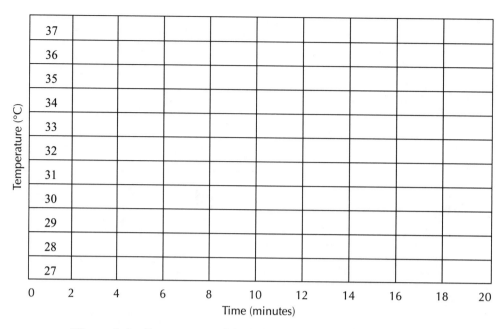

Figure 4-4   Temperature of the left hand (bare vs. covered) vs. time.

LABORATORY EXERCISE 5: PHYSIOLOGICAL RESPONSES TO INDIRECT HEAT

BACKGROUND AND THEORY

The application of therapeutic heat has been discussed in the previous laboratory exercise in terms of its therapeutic effects and the mechanisms involved in the vasodilation resulting from direct, mild heating procedures. However, individuals with circulatory impairments would not benefit from direct application of heat. If the transient tissue temperature rise occurred too rapidly, the blood could not remove the energy quickly enough due to impaired blood flow. If the temperature rise was too extreme, local arterial vessels could go into spasm and vasoconstrict, thereby closing the associated capillaries and depriving the tissue of oxygen. This would result in severe burns. An alternative to direct local heating is indirect heating in which the hypothalamus receives warm blood and reflexively causes systemic vasodilation to dissipate the heat and maintain core temperature. Reflex heating, indirect vasodilation, contralateral reflex response, consensual reaction, and indirect heating refer to the same phenomenon of heating the skin at a site that does not have a circulatory impairment, producing vasodilation and increased blood flow to that area and, additionally, increasing blood flow to the contralateral extremity (but to a lesser degree). The reflex response is dependent upon the intensity of the heat source and the area of skin affected directly by the heat. The reflex response is therefore proportional to the neural input at the site of temperature elevation.

The concept of reflex heating is not recent. As early as 1932, Gibbon and Landis demonstrated vasodilation occurring in the lower extremities in response to immersion of the forearm in warm water.[1] In 1949, Kerstake and Cooper demonstrated vasodilation in the forearm by measuring blood flow in response to heating the trunk.[2] They concluded that the latency period before vasodilation occurred was too short to be any other mechanism but reflex phenomenon.

Vasodilation produced by the direct application of heat occurs as a result of a local tissue temperature rise (TTR). The local TTR causes cell metabolism to increase and histamine to be released. The presence of histamine and metabolites causes relaxation of the vascular smooth muscle and subsequently vasodilation. Conversely, indirect methods of heating produce a systemic vasodilation. Indirect heating causes an increase in core (body) temperature. An increase in core temperature triggers the hypothalamus to send signals to the vasculature along sympathetic fibers. The ultimate goal of the hypothalamus is to produce vasodilation as a means of dissipating heat and decreasing core temperature. The hypothalamus can send out signals to withdraw sympathetic tone on the vessels, i.e., "let go" of the vessels so they can dilate. This is referred to as passive vasodilation. However, the hypothalamus may also choose to activate sympathetic fibers to release a vasodilator substance. This is referred to as active vasodilation.

In response to an increase in core body temperature, the hypothalamus sends signals to the skin (effector organ) via sympathetic fibers. These sympathetic fibers innervate the vascular smooth muscle and endothelial cells lining the blood vessels. **Norepinephrine (NE)** is released from the nerve ending and binds to an alpha adrenergic receptor on the smooth muscle to produce tonic vasoconstriction. ATP is co-released with NE but has the opposite effect and can be thought of as a buffer to the NE induced vasoconstriction. The hypothalamus can signal the release of adenosine from the adrenergic nerve endings. Adenosine binds to its receptor on the endothelial cell to stimulate the release of **nitric oxide (NO).** NO then directly effects the vascular smooth muscle and causes vasodilation. Under conditions of indirect heating the active vasodilatory response is turned on (by the hypothalamus) in order to facilitate the removal of heat to maintain core body temperature.

This laboratory exercise will demonstrate indirect heating by incorporating the use of hydrocollator packs (hot packs), the paraffin bath, a luminous heat source, and the whirlpool, all methods of superficial heating. The luminous heat source will be the same as that used in Laboratory Exercise 4. Hydrocollator packs are composed of a canvas bag with pockets; the pockets are filled with silica gel. The silica gel can absorb and hold a large amount of water; therefore, the hot pack expands when immersed in warm water. The packs are stored in a thermostatically controlled tank filled with water (71.1°–79.4°C). Hot packs are not applied directly to the exposed area; a layer of terrycloth about 3cm thick is placed between the hot pack and the individual's skin. Heat travels by conduction from the hot pack to the subject. The amount of heat flowing (H) through the body is represented by the following equation,

$$b_0 = \frac{\Sigma y - b\Sigma x}{n}$$

where k is thermal conductance, A is the area through which it flows, t is the time, T is the temperature gradient, and L is the thickness of the layer across which the temperature gradient is measured. The equation is of practical importance; for example, increasing the layer of towels (L) will decrease the flow of heat while wet towels will increase the thermal conductivity (k) and therefore increase the flow of heat. As with infrared heating, the appearance of mottling signals that the heat application should be discontinued. Hydrocollator packs are probably the most common form of superficial heating used, particularly for the relief of pain from secondary muscle spasm as well as the relief of abdominal and menstrual cramping.

The paraffin bath consists of a heated mixture of solid paraffin and paraffin or mineral oil, 6:1 ratio. The bath is kept in a thermostatically controlled metal container (51.7°–54.4°C). The paraffin bath has been used in the clinic longer than the hot pack for alleviating pain associated with chronic orthopedic lesions, such as rheumatoid and osteoarthritis (degenerative joint diseases) involving joints distal to the elbow or the knee. The methods for applying paraffin include dipping, immersion, and brushing. Dipping requires 8–12 consecutive immersions of the limb in the paraffin bath in order to form a thick glove of solid paraffin. The treated area is then wrapped in plastic, overwrapped with towels, and left for 10–20 minutes. The immersion method requires at least four preliminary dips to form a thin glove; the limb is then left immersed in the paraffin for 20–30 minutes. Paraffin can also be applied by brushing the area with eight to ten coats of paraffin, followed by wrapping of the area with towels and left alone for 10–20 minutes.

Hydrotherapy, i.e., whirlpool, is available for individuals with joint pain, open wounds, burns, or venous stasis ulcers. It is an effective agent for heating because water has a high specific heat and the buoyancy property of water makes it a useful therapy for exercise. However, caution must be taken with individuals who are edematous, have surgical wounds, or are pregnant. The Hubbard tank is one variation of the whirlpool; it allows whole body immersion and room for all four extremities to be exercised. Smaller whirlpools exist for upper and lower extremities.

Materials

paraffin bath, whirlpool, hydrocollator packs (hot packs), blankets
timers, surface thermometers, rectal thermocouples

Student Objectives

1. To observe the phenomenon of indirect heating.
2. To become familiar with the application of therapeutic heat with six different methods commonly utilized in clinics.
3. To plot the surface temperature change of the contralateral extremity for each student and determine which heating modality caused greater indirect heating.

STEP 1: EXPERIMENTAL PROCEDURES

The purpose of this laboratory exercise is to demonstrate indirect heating utilizing several different methods of superficial heating.

Paraffin Bath

Immersion method. The subject should sit with his or her leg hanging over the edge of the plinth such that the left leg can be lowered into the paraffin bath up to the tibial plateau. Remember to dip the leg at least four times before leaving the leg immersed in the bath for 30 minutes.

Dip and wrap method The subject should sit with his or her leg hanging over the edge of the plinth such that the left leg can be lowered into the paraffin bath up to the tibial plateau. The left leg should be dipped between eight and twelve times. Place a plastic bag or paper towels around the paraffin glove and wrap the leg in towels for insulation. The leg should remain wrapped for 30 minutes.

Whirlpool. The subject should sit at the edge of the plinth with his or her left leg, up to the tibial plateau, immersed in the water bath of 37–42°C, for 30 minutes.

Hot packs (hydrocollator packs). The subject should be sitting; place three hot packs (stored at 65°C) between three layers of toweling on the left foot for 30 minutes. If the hot pack was stored at 90°C, then six layers of toweling should be used between the skin and hot pack.

Infrared lamp. Subject should be supine on the plinth. Align the heat source at the appropriate angles to the left foot, according to the Inverse Square and Cosine Laws. Heat for 30 minutes. Towels may be placed over the exposed area if the heat becomes uncomfortable to the student.

1. Divide the class into five groups. Two volunteers are required from each group. Both students will experience the same method of heat application; however, one student will serve as the control model and the other student will be the experimental model. The student involved in the experimental procedure will have blankets draped over him or her to exaggerate the indirect heating response.

2. Core body temperature is to be recorded in addition to surface temperature. Each student will be given a thermocouple which will be inserted into the rectum to obtain body temperature. This method is more accurate and sensitive to small temperature changes than the oral thermometer. However, if students are unable or unwilling to use a rectal thermocouple, an oral thermocouple is acceptable.

3. To elicit the indirect heating response, Group I will use the paraffin bath-immersion technique, Group II will use the paraffin bath (dip and wrap) technique, Group III will use the whirlpool, Group IV will use hot packs, and Group V will use the IR lamp. Blankets should be draped over the experimental subject (upper body and lower extremities) to enhance the reflex response. Once the control or experimental subject is in his or her proper position, place the surface thermometer on the dorsal portion of the left foot.

4. Each student should assume responsibility for a portion of the experiment, i.e., set up of the procedure, reading skin temperature, recording results, monitoring subject for discomfort or pain, controlling and maintaining the temperature of the source.

5. Group I should begin timing for 30 minutes following the seven preliminary dips. Group II should start timing once the leg is wrapped. Group III can start once the water has reached 43°C. Group IV should begin timing for 30 minutes once the hot packs are in place. Group V should begin timing once the luminous source is turned on.

6. In five-minute intervals, record skin temperature measurements on Table 5-1 and core body temperature measurements on Table 5-2. Complete Table 5-3 as well.

7. Plot the **change** in skin temperature (initial temperature subtracted from the temperature at time of measurement) on Figure 5-1.

8. Plot the **change** in body temperature on Figure 5-1 but use different symbols to indicate body temperature.

Discussion Questions

1. Which subject, control or experimental, would you expect to have a greater increase in skin temperature? In core temperature? Why?

2. Was there a difference in the temperature change (surface and core) between the control and experimental subject as a result of heat application?

3. Did one heat modality produce a greater temperature increase than the others? Do all of the methods of heating penetrate to the same depth?

Table 5-1 Skin temperature measurements from the right foot of control (*C*) and experimental (*E*) students.

Time (min)		Temp (°C) Group I	Temp (°C) Group II	Temp (°C) Group III	Temp (°C) Group IV	Temp (°C) Group V
Initial	C					
	E					
5	C					
	E					
10	C					
	E					
15	C					
	E					
20	C					
	E					
25	C					
	E					
30	C					
	E					

Table 5-2 Body temperature measurements from control (*C*) and experimental (*E*) students.

Time (min)		Temp (°C) Group I	Temp (°C) Group II	Temp (°C) Group III	Temp (°C) Group IV	Temp (°C) Group V
Initial	C					
	E					
5	C					
	E					
10	C					
	E					
15	C					
	E					
20	C					
	E					
25	C					
	E					
30	C					
	E					

Table 5-3   Observations of control and experimental subjects.

	Group I C E	Group II C E	Group III C E	Group IV C E	Group V C E
Onset of sweating					
Subject perceives heat					
Subject feels discomfort					
Other comments					

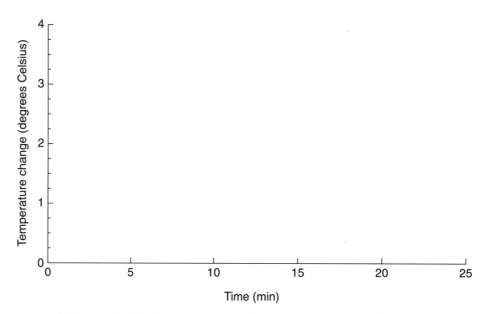

Figure 5-1   Plot the temperature change in non-treated limb of control (modality only) and experimental (modality with blanket) subjects. Using different symbols, plot the change in core temperature for both subjects.

NOTES

1. Gibbon and Landis, "Vasodilation in Lower Extremity in Response to Immersion of the Forearm in Warm Water", 1019–1036.
2. Kerstake and Cooper, "Vasodilation in the Forearm in Response to Heating the Trunk," 24.

LABORATORY EXERCISE 6: PHYSIOLOGICAL RESPONSES TO CRYOTHERAPY

BACKGROUND AND THEORY

The analgesic nature of cold application makes it a commonly prescribed treatment at home and in the clinic. Cold application by way of a cold pack, immersion in melting ice water, or ice massage is performed to reduce muscle tone (spasm), a secondary condition of underlying joint or skeletal pathology. Muscle spasms are continuous involuntary contractions which occur to immobilize and protect the injured area. However, muscle spasms ultimately create ischemia due to the contracting muscle compressing the intramuscular blood vessels. Cold decreases nerve conduction velocity, attenuates muscle spindle firing and slows muscle fiber contraction to reduce muscle spasm. Cold application is also used for individuals with upper motor lesions to reduce clonus and resistance to stretch so that further physical therapy programs can be performed.

The treatment of soft tissue injuries, i.e., sprain, includes the application of cold. A reduction in blood flow and edema are produced with cold application by vasoconstriction of the superficial arteries and capillaries. Mobility, elevation, and compression are also included in the treatment of acute soft tissue injuries. Laboratory Exercise 12 describes the effectiveness of this treatment in detail. Local vasoconstriction occurs immediately in the cooled area; general vasoconstriction occurs by reflex action of the central nervous system to conserve heat which is mediated by the cooler blood activating the hypothalamus. Once the temperature drops to 15°C, vasodilation occurs due to a reduction in sympathetic vasoconstrictor activity. Vasodilation, as seen by erythema (reddening of the area), protects local tissues from the damaging effects of maintaining such low temperatures. The physiological effects of cold application include a reduction in blood flow due to arteriole vasoconstriction and a decrease in metabolism as a result of low temperatures. A 10° decrease in temperature will reduce the rate of chemical reactions by one-half.

The depth of penetration of the cold stimulus is limited to 1.0–3.0 cm below the skin; if there is less than 1 cm of subcutaneous fat the temperature change can be seen 2 cm into the muscle. Cold penetrates deeper than heat due to a longer wavelength. If the area contains greater than 2 cm of fat, the depth of temperature change in the muscle is only 1 cm. To decrease the intramuscular temperature, the cold application must continue for a minimum of 20 minutes. The average temperature change in the skin, subcutaneous tissue, and muscle is seen in Figure 6-1.

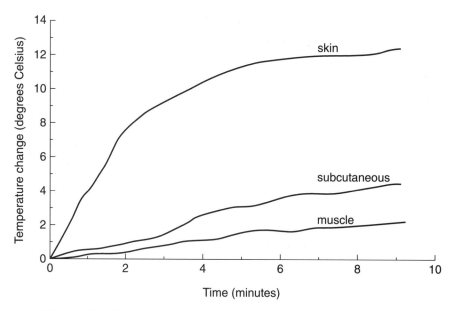

Figure 6-1 Temperature change in skin, muscle, and subcutaneous tissue of an individual with less than 1 cm of subcutaneous fat during ice application of the thigh.

The analgesic effect of cold application is achieved directly with the elevation of the pain threshold as a result of reducing the temperature on nerve fibers and receptors. It has been suggested that cold impulses bombard the cutaneous receptors and eventually override the pain receptors, thereby reducing the sensation of pain. Additionally, cold application reduces nerve conduction velocity. Indirectly, pain relief is attained with cold in the alleviation of muscle spasm and inflammation. The following exercise will involve the proper application of cold for therapeutic purposes, as well as determine how cold alters chronaxie, rheobase, a monosynaptic reflex (patellar tendon, knee jerk), and the H-reflex.

Materials

electrical stimulator, surface electrodes, cold packs
reflex hammer, EMG recording equipment

Student Objectives

1. To be familiar with the procedure of cold application using a cold pack.
2. To compare the chronaxie and rheobase values obtained during cold application with normal values.
3. To understand the difference between a monosynaptic reflex and the H-reflex.
4. To observe how cold influences a monosynaptic reflex and the H-reflex.

STEP 1: EXPERIMENTAL PROCEDURES

Chronaxie and rheobase are used to assess nerve and muscle integrity. Review Laboratory Exercise 2: Reliability includes a complete description of the two measurements in Step 2.

Divide the class into three main groups with at least three people in each group. Each group will be responsible for completing Steps 1, 2, and 3 to determine the effect of cold on chronaxie and rheobase values, a monosynaptic reflex, or the H-reflex. Only ONE student from each group will have measurements determined (chronaxie, rheobase, H-reflex, or monosynaptic reflex). However, that student will be evaluated twice, the first trial WITHOUT the use of cold packs and the second trial WITH the addition of cold packs. In this manner, we can assess the effect of cold on one individual's chronaxie and rheobase values, the H-reflex, or a monosynaptic reflex.

Chronaxie and Rheobase

1. One student will serve as both the control and experimental subjects for the experiment.
2. Subject should be supine on the plinth with the right leg exposed.
3. Place the dispersive electrode beneath the contralateral gastrocnemius muscle.
4. Locate the boundaries of the tibialis anterior muscle by having the subject invert and dorsiflex his or her ankle. The region midway between the distal and proximal muscle attachments will be the region in which the largest contraction can be observed.
5. Stimulate this region at various points to locate the point which produces the greatest contraction with the least amount of current.
6. Shave this region; apply conductive paste and a surface electrode.
7. To begin the strength-duration curve, set current intensity of the generator to zero and pulse width at 300 msec.
8. Gradually increase the current intensity until a minimal visible contraction is seen, i.e., the lowest current that produces a visible contraction. Record the current intensity on Table 6-1.
9. Repeat steps 7 and 8 for each pulse width listed in Table 6-1.
10. Plot the current strength (intensity) required to elicit the minimal visible contraction for each duration on Figure 6-2. Determine rheobase and chronaxie values. Rheobase (mV or mA) will be the intensity of current required to elicit the minimal visible contraction at the pulse width 300 msec. Find the pulse width (duration) on the strength-duration curve which corresponds to the current strength of twice the rheobase. The duration of the pulse is your chronaxie value (msec).
11. Place a cold pack wrapped in a moist towel on the student's right leg.
12. Repeat steps 7 through 10 after at least 10 minutes of cold application.
13. Compare chronaxie and rheobase points under control and cryotherapy treated conditions.

Table 6-1 Values obtained for construction of the strength-duration curve.

Pulse duration (msec)	Current without cold	(mV or MA) with cold	Comments
100			
70			
50			
30			
10			
7			
5			
3			
2			
1			
0.8			
0.6			
0.4			
0.3			
0.1			
.05			
Rheobase			
Chronaxie			

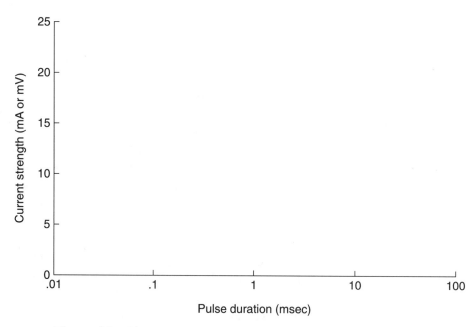

Figure 6-2 Plot strength duration curve under control and cryo-therapy treated conditions.

STEP 2:   THE MONOSYNAPTIC REFLEX

The patellar tendon reflex is an example of a **monosynaptic reflex** (Figure 6-3). The monosynaptic reflex is the simplest type of reflex, consisting of an **afferent** neuron transmitting impulses to the spinal cord, and an **efferent** neuron which sends impulses to the effector organ. The afferent neuron synapses directly with the efferent neuron in the spinal cord. By tapping the patellar tendon, the muscle **spindle** of the quadriceps is stretched. Stretching of the muscle spindle excites group **1a afferent** fibers which send impulses to the dorsal root of the spinal cord. A branch of the 1a afferent travels directly to the anterior horn of the gray matter in the spinal cord synapsing on the **alpha motor neuron (efferent neuron).** The alpha motor neuron innervates the quadriceps, causing the muscle to contract. The reflex ultimately causes the knee to extend; therefore, you may see the patellar tendon reflex also referred to as the knee jerk or stretch extensor reflex.

Eliciting the Patellar Tendon Reflex

This exercise is designed to study the effects of temperature on the patellar tendon reflex by cooling the thigh. This exercise will also demonstrate the inhibitory influence of the brain on the patellar tendon reflex (Figure 6-4).

1. The student should sit on the edge of a plinth and let his or her legs hang freely.
2. Palpate the tendon just below the knee; tap it with the reflex hammer or the side of your hand.

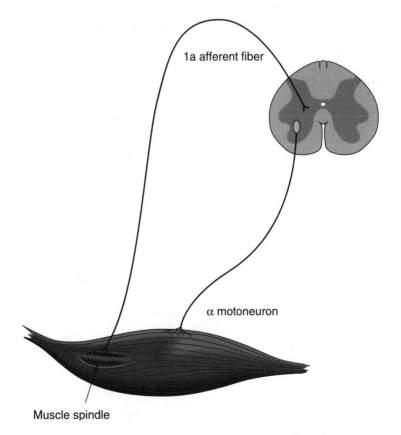

1a afferent fiber

α motoneuron

Muscle spindle

Figure 6-3   Neural circuit of a monosynaptic reflex.

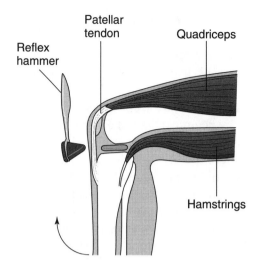

Tapping the tendon causes the lower
leg to swing up or extend.

Figure 6-4

3. Place the reference electrodes 2 cm proximal to the site of the tendon tap.
4. The muscle response should be assembled such that a hard copy of the EMG activity can be obtained.
5. The subject should close his or her eyes while another student elicits the reflex. A third student should be in charge of the EMG recording.
6. Apply a cold pack wrapped in a moist towel over the student's quadriceps. After 10 minutes, repeat the tendon tap.
7. Record observations in Table 6-2.

Point of Interest

To provide smooth, coordinated movements, muscles work in pairs. An agonist muscle performs the primary movement, i.e., biceps brachii contracts, allowing you to flex the elbow. The antagonist muscle performs the opposite action of the agonist. The antagonist muscle, in this case the triceps, when contracted, causes extension of the elbow. If the action of the antagonist muscle was not involved, then flexing the elbow would be a rapid, jerky movement. The quadriceps extensor muscles are the agonist muscles providing extension of the knee while the antagonists are the flexor muscles (hamstrings). In addition to the monosynaptic reflex neural pathway, the patellar tendon reflex also involves a branch of the 1a afferents synapsing on inhibitory interneurons. Inhibitory interneurons inhibit the alpha motor neuron activity to the antagonist flexor muscles. The inhibitory signals prevent the antagonist muscle from contracting to ensure that the agonist can contract maximally.

Table 6-2 Reflex response under control and experimental conditions.

	Time (elicit reflex to EMG activity)	Peak EMG activity
Reflex (control)		
Reflex (cold application)		

STEP 3:   THE HOFFMAN REFLEX

The Hoffmann or H-reflex is a reflex twitch of the gastrocnemius muscle which is elicited by electrically stimulating the tibial nerve located in the popliteal fossa. Tapping the Achilles tendon mechanically elicits a monosynaptic reflex twitch of the gastrocnemius called the Achilles tendon reflex (ATR). Be aware that the H-reflex and the Achilles tendon reflex are not the same. They both produce a twitch in the gastrocnemius; however, they do so through slightly different neural mechanisms.

The Hoffmann Reflex involves submaximal electrical stimulation of the **1a afferent** fibers from the muscle spindle in order to test the **alpha motoneuron excitability.** Upon electrical stimulation of the tibial nerve to produce the H-reflex (Figure 6-5), the 1a afferents are excited, transmit the impulse to the spinal cord, and monosynaptically synapse with the alpha motor neurons. Excitation of the alpha motor neuron will send the impulse to the gastrocnemius and cause muscle contraction. The result (muscle contraction) is the same response achieved by eliciting the Achilles tendon reflex. However, eliciting the muscle response by electrical stimulation bypasses the muscle spindle because the electrical stimulus acts directly on the 1a afferent fibers. Electrical stimulation of the tibial nerve also produces an **M-response.** The M-response is a muscle response occurring before the H-reflex, due to direct stimulation of motor axons in the tibial nerve (the nerve contains motor and sensory fibers).

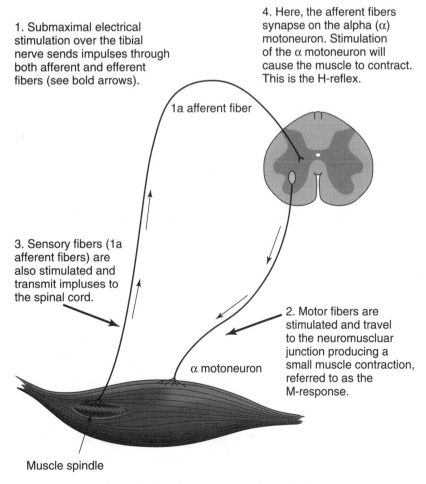

1. Submaximal electrical stimulation over the tibial nerve sends impulses through both afferent and efferent fibers (see bold arrows).

4. Here, the afferent fibers synapse on the alpha (α) motoneuron. Stimulation of the α motoneuron will cause the muscle to contract. This is the H-reflex.

1a afferent fiber

3. Sensory fibers (1a afferent fibers) are also stimulated and transmit impulses to the spinal cord.

2. Motor fibers are stimulated and travel to the neuromuscluar junction producing a small muscle contraction, referred to as the M-response.

α motoneuron

Muscle spindle

Figure 6-5   Neural circuit of the H-reflex.

In summary, the motor axons participating in the M-response are not involved in the H-reflex. The impulse does not travel to the muscle spindle to initiate a reflex contraction as with the knee jerk or Achille's tendon reflex; therefore, the number of motor units excited does not depend on the sensitivity of the muscle spindle to stretch. The strength of the electrical stimulation and the excitability of alpha motoneurons determines the amplitude of the H-response, whereas the sensitivity of the muscle spindle to stretch and the alpha motoneuron excitability determine the amplitude of the Achilles tendon reflex. In this laboratory we will be eliciting only the H-reflex to determine the effects of cold on the response.

Eliciting the H-Reflex

1. Student should be prone with right foot and ankle held at right angle off the edge of the plinth. There exists a specially designed apparatus which holds the ankle at a right angle; however, you may just use books or other material to secure the ankle and foot.

2. The anode should be soaked in saline and strapped over the posterior thigh.

3. Using a probe electrode in the approximate area of the tibial nerve, find the region which elicits the greatest maximum H-response with low voltage. Anchor the surface electrode (cathode) at that point.

4. Place the recording electrodes 2 cm proximal to the site of the tendon tap.

5. Position the ground electrode over the medial malleolus.

6. The muscle response should be assembled such that a hard copy of the EMG activity can be obtained.

7. To elicit the H-reflex, stimulate the tibial nerve with 0.1 msec rectangular wave pulse from stimulator. Gradually decrease the stimulus and observe the M-wave and H-response. If the M-wave amplitude decreases while the H-response remains constant, the H-reflex is confirmed.

8. Repeat step 7 with a cold pack wrapped in a moist towel on the student's lower right leg (calf).

9. Plot the EMG activity for control and cryotherapy H-reflexes on Figure 6-6. Compare the H-reflex obtained under control conditions with the H-reflex obtained with cryotherapy. Are the latency and amplitude the same?

STEP 4:   THE EFFECTS OF COLD ON SENSORY NEURONS

This exercise is designed to examine the effects of cold on blood flow by grasping ice in the right hand and recording the temperature and color changes in both hands. The sensitivity of the skin neurons will also be examined by performing two-point and coin discrimination tests before and after cold application.

1. Divide the class into a group of subjects and a group of experimenters.

2. Using the two-point threshold device, measure the two-point discrimination abilities of the subjects. The open right hand of the subject should lie on the table with the palm up. The eyes of the subject are to be closed. The experimenter will lightly touch the center of the subject's palm with the two-point

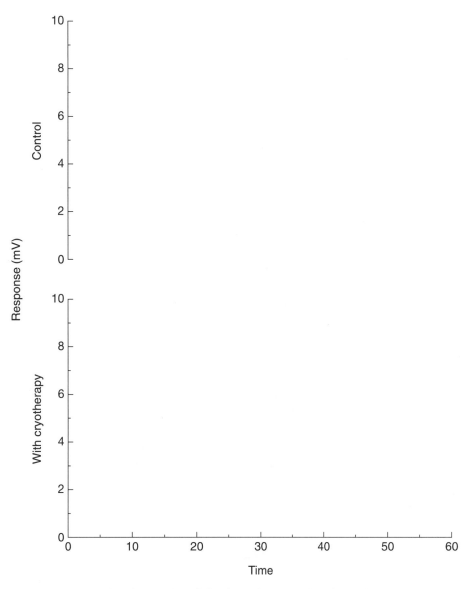

Figure 6-6   Plot the EMG activity from the control and cryotherapy treated H-reflexes.

discrimination device while the subject responds with the words "one" or "two," describing what was felt. The experimenter begins with the pins set for no space between them and gradually increases the distance by 1 mm each time until the subject responds with a "two." Record measurements on Table 6-3.

3. While the subject's eyes are still closed, a coin discrimination test will be given. The experimenter will place four coins (penny, nickel, dime, and quarter) in random order one at a time on the subject's palm. The subject will then guess which coin it is. Before administering the test, permit one practice trial in which the subject is allowed to guess the coins and is then given the correct answer. The practice trial will acquaint the subject with the feeling of the coins. Record the number of correct responses obtained in the real test on Table 6-3.

Table 6-3 Comparison of skin neuron sensitivity with discrimination tests before and after the application of ice.

	Before ice	After ice
Two-point discrimination (mm)		
Coin accuracy (number correct)		

4. Pair up an observer with a subject and have the experimenter record a description of the color of BOTH hands of the subject in Table 6-4.

5. With the right hand, the subject should grasp a handful of crushed ice, holding his or her hand over the bucket so the ice doesn't drip on the floor. After 2, 5, 10, and 15 minutes, the data recorder should note the appearance and surface temperature of both hands on Table 6-4. The ice should be replaced after each recording point or if it melts before the end of the test. During the experiment, the data recorder should report any sensations which the subject is feeling.

6. After 20 minutes, repeat the two-point and coin discrimination tests. Have the experimenter record answers in Table 6-3. Have the subject apply pressure on the cold hand with his or her warm hand and the data recorder note the changes, take a final surface temperature, and record. The data recorder should then graph the surface temperature of both hands on the same graph, using a solid line for the cold hand and a dashed line for the warm hand.

Anaslysis

1. How did the appearance of the hands change over time?
2. What changes occurred in the warm hand? Why?
3. What do the temperature changes show?
4. Why does the hand go numb?
5. What differences are noted in two-point discrimination before and after the experiment?
6. What occurs when pressure is applied to the cold hand?

Table 6-4 Temperature changes and observations of right and left hands during the application of ice.

	Temperature		Observations	
Time	Left hand	Right hand	Left hand	Right hand
0 min				
2 min				
5 min				
10 min				
15 min				

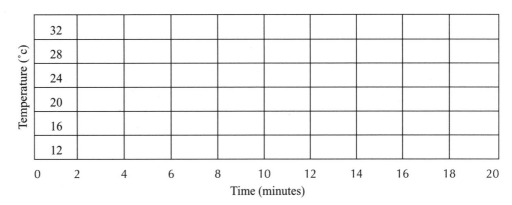

Figure 6-7   Right vs. left hand temperature.

⟫ *Point of Interest*

The instructor must emphasize the importance of standardizing the amount of force that is used while performing the tendon tap to assess tendon reflexes. The instructor may choose to point out that without standardization, the measured EMG signal may be totally random. The instructor may choose to design practice sessions where the students practice tendon taps multiple times with feedback to consistently achieve a criterion force. This can be achieved by tapping an input device on a dynamometer.

LABORATORY EXERCISE 7:   EXPERIMENTS AND DEMONSTRATIONS OF ELECTROTHERAPY

BACKGROUND AND THEORY

In order to appreciate the value of electrical stimulation for therapeutic purposes, we need to briefly review the physics of electrical currents and nerve and muscle physiology.

Tissues of the body are conductors of electricity because fluids bathing the tissues contain positive and negative ions (electrolytes). Movement of the ions through the fluid causes current to flow. The greater the number of electrolytes in solution, the greater the conductivity of that fluid. For example, muscles provide excellent conduction; however, tendons are more dense and do not conduct electricity well. Fat tissue is an insulator against electrical conduction and is therefore a poor conductor.

Across the membrane of all cells, an electrical potential exists. Negative ions accumulate on the surface inside the cell and an equal number of positive ions accumulate on the outer surface of the cell membrane, resulting in a potential difference across the membrane (Figure 7-1).

The difference in charge between the inside and outside of the cell membrane is the **membrane potential.** The membrane potential develops as a result of ions diffusing down their concentration gradient and active transport of ions across the membrane. Both processes result in a difference in the relative number of positive and negatively charged ions inside and outside the cell. The main determinant of the membrane potential is the K^+ ion's electrochemical gradient (see Figure 7-2 for movement of ions across membrane). However, the membrane potential is the combined equilibrium point of all the ions involved, such as Na^+, K^+, Ca^{2+}, and Cl^-. The **resting membrane potential** (RMP) or the difference in charge across the membrane under resting conditions, is established when the electrochemical gradients across the membrane of all of the ions involved are in balanced equilibrium. At this point there is no net flow of current, only a steady potential. The average RMP lies between 70–90 mV. RMP is usually written as -70 to -90 mV because the inside of the cell is negative with respect to the outside. The two most important ions in setting up the RMP are potassium (K^+) and sodium (Na^+). K^+ is in greater concentration inside the cell while sodium is in greater concentration outside the cell. The membrane contains protein channels through which sodium and potassium ions leak according to their concentration gradient, i.e., Na^+ leaks in, K^+ leaks out. The channels are more permeable ($100\times$) to potassium than sodium. The

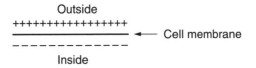

Figure 7-1

Na$^+$/K$^+$ pump maintains the RMP by driving 3 Na$^+$ ions out of the cell for every 2 K$^+$ ions into the cell to preserve the electrochemical gradients of Na$^+$ and K$^+$. Consequently, more positive ions are constantly pumped out of the cell, leaving the inside more negative with respect to the outside of the cell.

Now that we are aware that cells 'hum' with electrical activity generated by movement of ionic currents through ion pumps and channels, what events occur at the membrane that cause an impulse to travel down a nerve or a muscle? In other words, how can an impulse or **action potential** be elicited and what changes occur in the membrane? Any mechanical, electrical, or chemical disruption of the membrane that causes sodium to diffuse into the cell (increases sodium conductance) could elicit an action potential. The action potential can be divided into three stages, Figure 7-3. The resting stage consists of the resting membrane potential prior to initiation of the action potential. The membrane is **polarized** at this stage, -90mV. **Depolarization,** the second stage, occurs due to a sudden increase in the membrane potential. An increase refers to the membrane potential becoming more positive or the inside of the cell becoming more positive. Essentially, the charge across the membrane reverses (depolarizes) and the impulse or depolarization wave travels along the entire length of the nerve or muscle fiber. An appropriate stimulus (electrical, chemical, or mechanical) causing disruption of the membrane will activate voltage-gated sodium channels to open, i.e., as the voltage across the membrane becomes more positive and approaches zero, the channels open. Sodium will then follow its concentration gradient and flow into the cell, creating a positive charge inside the cell. Within a fraction of a second, the inactivation of sodium channels occur and potassium channels open, allowing potassium to flow down its concentration gradient out of the cell to re-establish the membrane potential. Rapid flux of potassium ions out of the cell characterizes **repolarization,** the third stage.

Action potentials can be elicited in nerve and muscle fibers. Generally, motor axons transmit the impulse to the muscle via a **neurotransmitter** to produce muscle contraction. An action potential travels along the nerve fiber to the **neuro-muscular junction** at the nerve terminal, Figure 7-4. The action potential causes the opening of sodium and calcium channels in the axonal membrane. Calcium flux

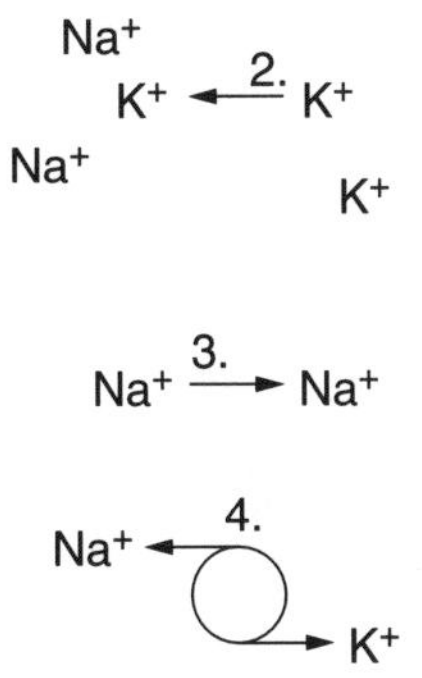

Na$^+$
   K$^+$ $\xleftarrow{\;2.\;}$ K$^+$
Na$^+$
                K$^+$
	1. Membrane is more permeable to potassium than sodium

	2. Potassium leaks out of the cell through protein channels according to its concentration gradient.
Na$^+$ $\xrightarrow{\;3.\;}$ Na$^+$	3. Sodium leaks into the cell through protein channels according to the concentration gradient.

Na$^+$ $\xrightarrow{\;4.\;}$
       $\bigcirc$
             $\searrow$ K$^+$
	4. Na$^+$–K$^+$ pump maintains the resting membrane potential by driving 3 Na$^+$ ions out of the cell for every 2 K$^+$ ions into the cell.

Figure 7-2   Movement of Na$^+$ and K$^+$ ions across the membrane.

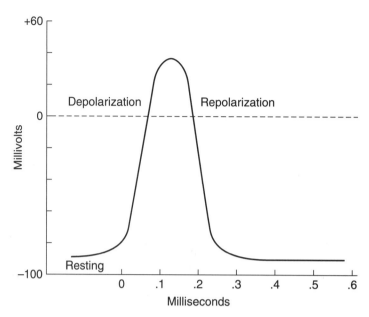

Figure 7-3   Three phases of an action potential.

into the nerve terminal causes vesicles which contain the neurotransmitter, **acetyl-choline (Ach),** to align along the inner surface of the membrane. The vesicles fuse with the membrane and exocytose, spilling Ach into the space between the nerve terminal and the surface of the muscle fiber, called the **synaptic cleft.** Ach binds to receptors on the muscle causing Na+ channels in the sarcolemma (muscle membrane) to open. Sodium flux into the membrane transmits the action potential to the muscle fiber. The electrical event of transmitting the impulse from the nerve to the muscle depends upon the Ach binding on the muscle, which ultimately depends on the amount of calcium flowing into the nerve terminal.

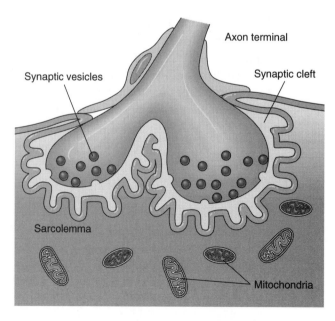

Figure 7-4   Neuromuscular junction.

The following steps occur within the muscle and are illustrated in Figures 7-5a and 7-5b. The action potential travels along the T-tubules of the muscle and causes calcium to be released from the sarcoplasmic reticulum. Calcium travels to nearby regions of actin and myosin (protein filaments which make up the contractile unit of a muscle fiber). The thin filament, actin, consists of two strands wrapped around each other like a rope, Figure 7-5b. In the groove between the two strands of actin lies another protein, **tropomyosin,** which acts to cover/uncover the binding site between actin and myosin. Attached to the tropomyosin is a fourth protein, **troponin,** which contains binding sites for calcium and ATP. As calcium binds to its site on troponin, a conformational change in tropomyosin occurs revealing the attachment site for the myosin. Myosin, the thick filament, contains extensions called **cross bridges,** which attach to the actin filaments. Under the appropriate conditions, the cross bridges will pull actin across the myosin filaments and generate a contraction. Cross bridge formation between the actin and myosin filaments requires the splitting of ATP on the myosin head of the cross bridge. Energy released during the breakdown of ATP is stored in the myosin head and used to pull actin across the myosin filaments once the cross bridge binds to the actin filament. This event is called the "power stroke," Figure 7-6. Once the power stroke is complete and a shortening contraction has occurred, ATP must bind to the myosin head in order to detach the cross bridge from actin. If ATP was not available to bind to the myosin head, cross bridges would not detach and the muscle would be in a state of rigor, i.e., rigor mortis. In addition to ATP binding, relaxation is dependent upon the uptake of Ca^{2+} back into the sarcoplasmic reticulum.

Nerve and muscle cells act as **capacitors** in the same way as capacitors exist in electrical circuits. By definition, capacitance refers to the ability to store electrical charge. Nerve and muscle cells have the ability to store charge (electrons) and

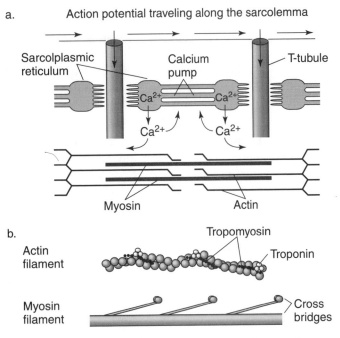

Figure 7-5 (a) Action potential traveling along the sarcolemma and (b) an enlarged view of the actin and myosin filaments.

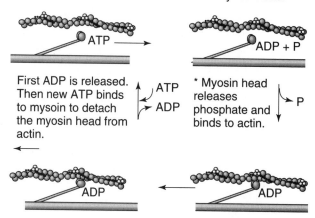

ATP bound to the mysoin head is cleaved to ADP and P, which remain bound to the myosin head.

First ADP is released. Then new ATP binds to mysoin to detach the myosin head from actin.

* Myosin head releases phosphate and binds to actin.

Myosin head undergoes a conformational change. This shifts the actin filament and generates force. It is referred to as the power stroke.

Figure 7-6   Events that occur during the "Power Stroke" of muscle contraction.

* Calcium binding to troponin is necessary to reveal the attachment site on the actin filament for myosin. Calcium binding to troponin causes a conformational change in tropomyosin. Tropomyosin shifts and reveals the actin-myosin binding site.

will discharge once they can no longer store charge. A coin analogy may be helpful in understanding the concept of capacitance (Figure 7-7).

If we filled the surfaces of a quarter and a dime with electrical charge, more charge and obviously more time would be required to fill the surface of the quarter. The quarter would be said to have a higher capacitance then the dime, i.e., it can store more charge and requires a longer time to discharge. With a smaller capacitance, the dime discharges more rapidly because its ability to store charge is less than the quarter. Nerve fibers can respond to a greater number of stimuli because they have a smaller capacitance than muscle fibers. Having a smaller capacitance, or ability to store charge, the nerve cell discharges and the current passes through the cell. Clinically, an individual with an intact nerve supply can respond to a greater number of stimuli than an individual with denervated muscles. Muscle fibers have a greater capacitance, and therefore require a longer duration or lower frequency of stimulation before the fiber will reach its capacity to store electrons and discharge. Nerve fibers can respond to a stimulus with frequency of 60 Hz. At lower frequencies, like the ones used to stimulate denervated muscle, nerve fibers may not depolarize because the fiber accommodates to the stimulus. **Accommodation** refers to

Quarter   Dime   **Figure 7-7**

the ability of the membrane to adjust its ion flow to maintain resting potential, in response to a low frequency stimulus. The stimulus may alter the membrane potential, but the rise in potential is so slow that the membrane adjusts to the new potential rather than eliciting an action potential. If denervated muscle lies deep, stimulation with a low frequency, direct current, will produce accommodation of superficial nerves and depolarization of muscle fibers. Generally if the time to go from zero to peak amplitude exceeds 10 msec, axon depolarization will not occur.

Therapeutic use of electrical current consists of applying an external stimulus to muscle or nerve to elicit muscle contraction or impulse, respectively. An **electrical current** is nothing more than a string of electrons (negatively charged particles) passing along a conductor (wire or nerve). **Current** intensity or flow is measured in amperes and is referred to as amperage. The electrical current encounters resistance along the conductor, much the same way as resistance is present in blood flow through the vessels. **Resistance** is measured in ohms. An **electromotor force** (EMF) is necessary for current to flow. The EMF provides the "push" for current to flow. The EMF is measured in volts and may be referred to as voltage. The relationship between current, resistance, and voltage can be expressed mathematically in the equation describing **Ohm's Law,** $i = v/R$, where i, v, and R represent current, voltage, and resistance, respectively. Ohm's Law states that current intensity is directly proportional to the voltage and indirectly proportional to the resistance.

The response to external nerve and muscle stimulation is governed by the **Law of Dubois Reymond.** The law states that the variation in current density, not the absolute density, acts as the stimulus to nerve or muscle. Therefore, when applying an external stimulus, the amplitude or intensity must be great enough to depolarize the membrane (nerve or muscle), the duration of the stimulus must be long enough for the action potential to spread, and the rate of change of voltage must be rapid enough to prevent accommodation from occurring.

Electrical current is represented in the form of waves with varying shape, amplitude, direction, and duration depending on the particular current chosen. **Direct current** (DC) refers to current which flows in one direction. The electrons travel from the negative pole to the positive pole. **Alternating current** (AC) reverses the direction of flow twice every cycle. Flow of electrons reverses directions because of a change in the polarity of the terminals within the generator. Compare AC and DC current in Figure 7-8. Alternating and direct current can be **continuous** or **modulated.** A continuous current has no change in its waveform, whereas a modulated current has a varying waveform due to interrupted or surged pulses.

Application of a continuously modulated *direct current* will cause a **twitch response** of the normally innervated muscle. The contractile response occurs at the completion of the electrical circuit and no further muscle response can occur because depolarization is maintained in the axons stimulated by the negative pole. At the positive pole, hyperpolarization occurs upon stimulation and is likewise maintained as long as DC current flows. The muscle cannot recover from depolarization (negative pole) or hyperpolarization (positive pole) and contract again until the energy flow ceases or changes directions. In contrast, a **tetanic response** is observed when stimulating normally innervated muscle with an *alternating current* of the same intensity but a frequency of 60 Hz or greater. The muscle contracts and remains contracted until the circuit is interrupted. It is important to realize that the sustained contraction is not due to each individual muscle fiber remaining contracted, but because muscle fibers are stimulated at different sites and contract independently. The change in voltage during the 60 Hz current cause a greater stimulus

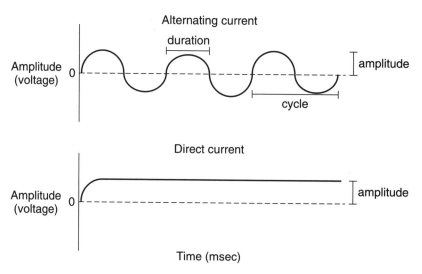

Figure 7-8   Comparison of alternating and direct currents.

response in the muscle. However, the response to the same current intensity and frequency in *denervated muscle* would differ. The varying responses of normally innervated and denervated muscle can be explained by comparing the capacitance of nerve and muscle fibers. Recall that the capacitance of muscle is larger than that of nerve fibers. At 60 Hz, the voltage fluctuations would be too rapid to allow for depolarization along the muscle fiber. Denervated muscle fibers require a frequency of 40 Hz or less to allow enough time for depolarization of the muscle membrane, generation of the muscle action potential, and muscle contraction. In addition, denervated muscle fibers will have only a twitch response regardless of the duration of current. Generally, axons require current flow in one direction for 0.1–1.0 msec, and denervated muscle fibers require current flow for 2.5–3.0 msec and up to 10 msec if the muscle has been deprived of nerve supply over one week.

> *If a muscle response (contraction) was observed with the use of a stimulating current on an individual with an intact peripheral nervous system, is the response due to depolarization of the muscle membrane directly or due to the depolarization of the motor nerves?*

> The response will always be the result of depolarization of the motor nerves because nerve fibers have a smaller capacitance than muscle fibers and will discharge sooner. Therefore, the smaller the capacity of the membrane, the less stimulus amplitude needed to cause depolarization.

Nerve and muscle stimulating devices can supply currents of varying characteristics in an attempt to stimulate nerve or muscle. The current may be of continuous, surge, or interrupted modulation, AC or DC type, and consist of frequencies in the range of 0 (DC only) to 3,000 Hz (AC and DC). The tissue can be excited by needle or surface electrodes. Electrodes vary in size and can be used in uni- or bipolar configuration and up to 10 electrodes may be used at once for nerve/muscle stimulation. The range of choices is vast due to the many different neurological, vascular, and orthopedic problems encountered in patients. Generally, *low voltage alternating currents* are more comfortable for the patient if a contractile response is desired. Direct currents may cause irritation below the electrodes due to the accumulation of positive ions (free hydrogen) below the cathode (negative terminal) and negative ions (free oxygen and acid) beneath the anode (positive terminal). Painful chemical reactions, acidic and alkaline buildup, develop below the electrodes and damage the skin. In addition, **hyperemia** (reddening) is commonly seen following use of continuous DC; DC is particularly uncomfortable for patients with intact sensory systems because of the intense stimulus to the cutaneous neurons. Alternating current, however, will not cause acidic or alkaline buildup beneath the electrodes as occurs with DC because the current flow reverses direction each one half cycle. A *high voltage direct current* is now available which does not cause significant skin irritation or visible hyperemia because it is delivered via paired sub-threshold pulses of extremely short duration (150 μsec). The success of obtaining a nerve or muscle response is dependent upon (1) the duration of current flow—i.e., it must be long enough in one direction to allow for depolarization of the membrane—and (2) the voltage—i.e., whether the voltage is high enough to cause depolarization of the membrane. The less excitable the membrane, the larger the capacitance (capacitance is the inverse of excitability) so the longer the stimulus current must flow or the higher the voltage necessary to elicit the response.

While the principles of electricity are the basis for all electrical stimulating devices, the applications of these devices vary from analgesia/pain management, strength training, and wound healing to functional electrical stimulation and iontophoresis (ion transfer through dermis). Although electrical stimulation has a variety of uses, equally important are the situations in which electrotherapy should not be used or should be used with caution. It is best to avoid electrical stimulation on individuals with pacemakers or other heart conditions. The spread of the current could interfere with the rhythm of the beating heart. However, with ECG monitoring, electrotherapy (i.e., TENS) has been performed on patients with pacemakers. Patients with thrombophlebitis should not have electrotherapy treatment, as well. Electrotherapy may facilitate the breaking away of thrombi from the blood vessel wall, which could lead to embolism. Electrodes should not be placed on abnormal areas of the skin, i.e., rash, psoriasis, abrasion. The current will concentrate in these areas and produce chemical burns in the underlying tissue.

This laboratory will not involve the use of any one specific electrical stimulating device or method. Instead, the exercises in this laboratory were designed to reinforce the principles of electrical current and the effect of applying an external stimulus to the body over a nerve or muscle.

Materials

surface electrodes (two sizes)
stimulating device which will deliver AC and DC
potato, potassium iodide, pH meter, litmus paper

Student Objectives

1. To describe the electrical events in the body which lead to nerve impulses and muscle contractions.
2. To compare the effects of two electrodes of different sizes.
3. To compare the effect of placing the active electrode in the negative or positive terminal.

4. To differentiate between the cathode and anode with a simple water test.
5. To differentiate between alternating and direct currents.

STEP 1: EXPERIMENTAL PROCEDURES

This exercise was designed around demonstrations which reinforce the basic principles of electricity, not on the application of one specific type of stimulating current.

Alternating and Direct Currents

Alternating and direct currents are available for use in the clinic. At the most basic level, the two currents differ in terms of the direction of current flow. An alternating current reverses the direction of electron flow twice each cycle. Conversely, a direct current consists of current flowing in one direction with a constant stimulus amplitude and infinitely long wavelength. The following demonstration will illustrate the difference between two currents of equal intensity, one AC and one DC, in their effect on the patient.

1. Divide class into groups of two or more students so that each group has a stimulating device, i.e., the number of available machines will determine the number of groups to divide into.
2. Apply two electrodes (at least 5 x 5 cm) anywhere on the student's body at an arbitrary distance, i.e., quadriceps, gastrocnemius. Remember to clean area with alcohol and then rub the area with a towel after the alcohol has evaporated to eliminate unnecessary skin impedance before placing the electrodes on the student. Attach electrodes to lead cords and attach lead cords to the stimulating device.
3. Set the stimulator to alternating current 60 Hz frequency, continuous modulation and zero intensity.
4. Increase the intensity to the student's tolerance. It is not necessary to elicit a muscle contraction.
5. Allow the current to flow for 5 minutes, adjusting the intensity according to the student's tolerance.
6. Record the voltage/amperage after 5 minutes. Reduce intensity to zero and remove electrodes. Inspect the skin and record any changes observed.
7. After 5 to 10 minutes, reapply new electrodes to the area adjacent to the first set of electrodes.
8. Set the stimulator to direct current, continuous modulation, and zero intensity.
9. Adjust the current intensity to the student's tolerance. Maintain the current flow for 5 minutes or as long as the student can tolerate the stimulus (whichever is the shortest). Record the final voltage/amperage before turning the intensity down to zero.
10. Remove electrodes and inspect the skin.

Discussion Questions

1. Which current was more tolerable for the student? Explain why.
2. Which current would be more effective to elicit muscle contraction?

3. Discuss the cause of hyperemia. What other situations would produce hyperemia? You may wait to answer this after completing Step 2.

STEP 2: COMPARE VOLTAGE NEEDED TO ELICIT MUSCLE CONTRACTION WITH ALTERNATING AND DIRECT CURRENTS

Remain in the same groups for the following exercises. There is a difference in the amount of voltage needed to elicit a contraction depending upon the type of current chosen. Consider the Law of Dubois Reymond to predict which current requires a greater voltage.

When applying a direct current, one electrode is always active or stimulating and one electrode is always inactive or dispersive. If a direct current were applied, predict whether the voltage required to elicit muscle contraction would be greater with a negative or positive stimulating electrode, using your knowledge of the resting membrane potential.

1. Decide, within the group, on which muscle group (i.e., quadriceps, gastrocnemius) to stimulate. Apply two electrodes over the muscle to be stimulated. Remember to clean area with alcohol and then rub the area with a towel after the alcohol has evaporated to eliminate unnecessary skin impedance. Attach electrodes to lead cords and attach lead cords to the stimulating device.
2. Set the stimulator to **alternating current** 60 Hz frequency, continuous modulation and zero intensity.
3. Increase the intensity to elicit a minimal visible contraction.
4. Record the minimum voltage/amperage necessary to elicit the contraction. Reduce intensity to zero and remove electrodes.
5. Apply new electrodes to the same muscle on the **opposite** limb.
6. Set the stimulator to **direct current,** continuous modulation and zero intensity.
7. Increase the intensity to elicit the minimal visible contraction.
8. Record the voltage/amperage necessary to obtain contraction.
9. Turn intensity down to zero and remove electrodes.
10. Reverse the polarity of the leads. Repeat steps 8–10.

Discussion Questions

1. Was your prediction of which current required a higher voltage correct?
2. Apply the Law of Dubois Reymond to what you observed.
3. Which electrode, positive or negative, requires the greater voltage when used as the stimulating electrode to obtain a muscle contraction? Explain this in terms of membrane polarity.

STEP 3: DEMONSTRATION OF ION MOVEMENT WITH DIRECT CURRENT

Using a potato and potassium iodide solution, we can demonstrate how a direct current causes ions to flow in one direction. Clinically, this concept is used to introduce drugs to a localized area. This is known as **iontophoresis.** The success of iontophoresis is based on the fact that like charges repel like charges. Introducing a drug with a positive charge will be effective if the drug is driven through the skin with the positive pole (anode). The positively charged drug will be repelled from the anode and consequently move through the skin into the subcutaneous tissue.

1. Divide the class into as many groups as there are DC generators. Each group needs one potato.
2. Cut a groove out of the potato (approximately in the middle). Fill the groove with potassium iodide solution. There should be a "lake" of iodide in the potato.
3. Place the anode in one end of the potato and the cathode in the opposite end.
4. Turn the generator on. Send a current of 40–50 mA through the potato.
5. Watch for any color changes in the potato. Cut the potato in various places to more clearly observe the results. Please explain.

STEP 4: DEMONSTRATION OF THE EVENTS OCCURRING AT THE POSITIVE AND NEGATIVE ELECTRODES USING DIRECT CURRENT

The following demonstration was included to further explain the irritating effects of using a continuously modulated direct current. You will need to fill a 200 ml beaker or similar clear container with saline.

1. Place metal terminals from the two lead cords in saline. Be sure that they are separated from each other. Plug terminals into the stimulating device with the intensity set at zero and direct current selected.
2. Increase the intensity to an arbitrary level, i.e., the intensity used in Step 1. Monitor pH at both terminals with a pH meter.
3. Observe the terminals in the water. You should see bubbles around the terminals due to the dissociation of water molecules. Which terminal has more bubbles? Place blue and pink litmus paper in the solution around each terminal. Record the color change on Table 7-1.
4. Decrease current intensity to zero. Turn stimulator off.

Discussion Questions

1. Why do more bubbles accumulate at one pole than the other?
2. Explain the results of the litmus test. Which ions accumulated at the negative pole and which ions accumulated at the positive pole? Why?

Table 7-1   Results of litmus test from the positive and negative terminals.

Color change	Positive terminal	Negative terminal
Blue litmus paper		
Pink litmus paper		

3. Is the chemical reaction which occurs with continuously modulated direct current necessary for action potential formation?

STEP 5:   *COMPARISON OF HIGH VOLT AND LOW VOLT STIMULATION*

The following exercise will demonstrate why high voltage stimulation is used even though only direct currents can deliver this type of stimulus. A high voltage direct current is available which does not cause significant skin irritation or visible hyperemia because it is delivered via paired sub-threshold pulses of extremely short duration (150 μsec).

1. Locate motor point of right gluteus maximus. Clean the area with alcohol and rub with a towel before applying a surface electrode. Place a large dispersive electrode on opposite glut or over bony surface.
2. Apply a high-volt stimulus to the area. Record duration of stimulus and voltage required to obtain a muscle contraction. Remove electrodes.
3. Locate motor point on left gluteus maximus. Prepare the area as before and apply a surface electrode. The dispersive electrode can be placed on the opposite glut or over a bony surface.
4. Apply a low voltage stimulus. Record the voltage and duration of stimulus required to obtain a muscle contraction. It is possible that a contraction will not be obtained before the student feels uncomfortable.

Discussion Questions

1. Compare the student's response to the two stimuli.
2. There is not one defined explanation for why the high voltage stimulus is more comfortable. How do the stimuli differ? (voltage? current?)
3. Did hyperemia or skin irritation occur?

STEP 6:   *ELECTRODE SIZE AND PLACEMENT*

This exercise will be more useful when you begin recording the electrical activity in the muscle. However, it is still applicable to nerve and muscle stimulation. Electrodes may be of varying size. Size plays a role in the intensity of current being delivered. For example, if your only two electrodes are of different sizes, the smaller electrode automatically becomes the active electrode and the large one becomes the inactive electrode. With high voltage stimulation, the standard electrode sizes are 500 cm^2 for the large dispersive electrodes and 1–65 cm^2 for the small active electrodes. The advantage of using a bipolar electrode set-up is that a greater concentration of energy per volume of tissue exists with more than one electrode which leads to a greater amount of energy reaching the muscle for a given current intensity. If the skin impedance is high or if denervation is apparent, bipolar electrode placement is more effective than a monopolar set-up. Of course, the smaller the concentration of energy per volume of tissue, the greater the patient comfort. By

Table 7-2   Current intensity required to elicit a minimal visible contraction (MVC) under the four conditions.

Electrode Size Placement	Intensity (mV or mA)
Large electrodes	
Small electrodes	
Adjacent electrodes	
Electrodes 5 cm apart	

increasing the distance between the two electrodes, the ratio of energy per volume tissue decreases, and accordingly so will any discomfort. Conduct the following experiments if you have a device (oscilloscope) to record compound action potentials of muscles (motor unit potentials).

1. Decide within your group on a muscle to stimulate.
2. Locate the motor point of the muscle. Place two large electrodes 2 cm apart over the surface of the muscle. Remember to clean the skin with alcohol and rub the surface with a dry towel prior to placing the electrodes on the skin.
3. Record the current intensity required to elicit a minimal visible contraction on Table 7-2.
4. Repeat steps 2 and 3 with small electrodes.
5. Locate the motor point of the muscle. Place two large electrodes next to each other over the muscle. Clean the skin with alcohol and rub the area with a dry towel prior to placing the electrodes on the skin.
6. Record the current intensity required to elicit a minimal visible contraction on Table 7-2.
7. Repeat steps 5 and 6 but place the electrodes 5 cm apart.

Discussion Questions

1. Was there a relationship between the intensity required to elicit a minimal visible contraction and the size of the electrodes?
2. What is the relationship between electrode placement and the intensity required to elicit a minimal visible contraction?

Answers to Exercise 7

STEP 1:   ALTERNATING AND DIRECT CURRENTS

1. The alternating current will be more tolerable than the direct current. Direct currents may cause irritation (acidic and alkaline buildup) below the electrodes and damage the skin. Hyperemia may exist following use of continuous DC. Also, DC is particularly uncomfortable for patients with intact

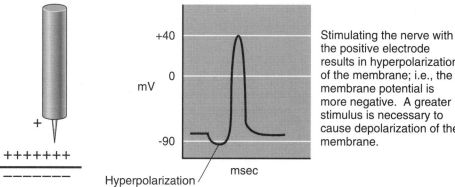

Stimulating the nerve with the positive electrode results in hyperpolarization of the membrane; i.e., the membrane potential is more negative. A greater stimulus is necessary to cause depolarization of the membrane.

Figure 7-9

sensory systems because of the intense stimulus to the cutaneous neurons. Alternating current, however, will not cause acidic or alkaline buildup beneath the electrodes or hyperemia as occurs with DC because the current flow reverses direction each one half cycle.

2. *Normal innervation:* The intensity required to elicit a muscle contraction is less with an AC than with DC.

   Denervation: DC could be applied to elicit muscle contraction by depolarizing the muscle fiber directly. Even though the current would be applied for a longer duration, the individual would not be in any discomfort because the muscle is denervated.

3. Hyperemia is a result of vasodilation. Cutaneous cells release histamine or histamine-like substances in response to the stimulating current. Histamine causes local vasodilation and thus, hyperemia.

STEP 2:   COMPARE VOLTAGE NEEDED TO ELICIT MUSCLE CONTRACTION WITH ALTERNATING AND DIRECT CURRENTS

1. Again, the DC requires a greater voltage than AC.

2. Law of Dubois Reymond states that not only must the amplitude and duration of current be sufficient to cause muscle contraction, but the change in voltage must be rapid to insure that accommodation does not occur.

3. A greater voltage is required when the positive electrode is the stimulating electrode. At rest, the membrane is positive outside with respect to the inside. Before depolarization occurs, there is hyperpolarization of the membrane, i.e., the membrane potential is more negative with the positive stimulating electrode (Figure 7-9).

STEP 3:   DEMONSTRATION OF ION MOVEMENT WITH DIRECT CURRENT

Color Change

Blue accumulation at the positive pole (anode) because it attracts the negatively charged iodide.

STEP 4:   DEMONSTRATION OF THE EVENTS OCCURRING AT THE POSITIVE AND NEGATIVE ELECTRODE USING DIRECT CURRENTS

1. Bubbles appear at both poles due to partial dissociation of water into H^+ and O^- ions. Hydrogen ions accumulate beneath the negative electrode. There are twice as many hydrogen ions, therefore twice as many bubbles accumulate beneath the negative pole.

2. The saline solution is made up of sodium chloride and water. With the passing of a direct current, the NaCl dissociates into Na^+ and Cl^- ions. Sodium ions will accumulate beneath the negative electrode and chloride ions will accumulate beneath the positive terminal initially. Secondary chemical reactions occur. Water dissociates into hydrogen ions (H^+) and hydroxide ions (OH^-). The sodium ions combine with hydroxide to form sodium hydroxide beneath the negative pole (cathode). Chloride ions combine with free hydrogen ions to form hydrochloric acid beneath the positive pole (anode). The results of the litmus test should be as follows: red at the positive pole indicating acidic solution, and blue at the negative terminal indicating a basic solution.

3. No, the reaction that occurs at the positive and negative poles with DC are not necessary to elicit muscle contraction.

STEP 5:   COMPARISON OF HIGH VOLT AND LOW VOLT STIMULATION

1. Compare the student's response to the two stimuli.

2. The high voltage generators deliver paired sub-threshold pulses which temporally sum to cause depolarization. High voltage generators are constant voltage rather than constant current as opposed to low voltage generators.

3. Hyperemia should not occur with the high voltage stimulator because the current is pulsed rather than continuous. The pulsed nature of the stimulus prevents the alkaline and acidic buildup beneath the electrodes.

STEP 6:   ELECTRODE SIZE AND PLACEMENT

1. Lesser intensity required to elicit a minimal visible contraction with smaller electrodes (the smaller the electrode the greater the stimulus for any given intensity).

2. Smaller intensity required to elicit a minimal visible contraction with electrodes closer together.

LABORATORY EXERCISE 8: MICE: HOW DOES IT WORK?

BACKGROUND AND THEORY

An acute soft tissue injury causes pain, edema, and loss of function. The primary goal of treatment is to reduce edema because this will alleviate pain and restore function. This laboratory exercise examines the mechanisms responsible for edema reduction during the treatment of a soft tissue injury.

The application of cold is probably the most universal treatment for an acute injury such as a sprain. The treatment also includes mobilizing of the joint *within the pain-free range of motion,* wrapping the injury to apply pressure, and elevating the area; the acronym for this procedure is **MICE** or **M**obilization, **I**ce, **C**ompression, and **E**levation. The following laboratory will not involve treating someone with a soft tissue injury. Instead, this exercise will concentrate on the physiological principles of how these four steps function to improve tissue nutrition based on Starling's Law of fluid flow across the capillary membrane. We know the steps in treating a sprain; let's look at why these steps are effective.

Inflammation occurs as a result of tissue injury. Inflammation consists of vasodilation of local blood vessels and therefore increased blood flow to the area. Increased capillary permeability occurs which permits large amounts of pure plasma to leak into the interstitial spaces, culminating in edema formation. Blood clotting is possible due to excess amounts of fibrinogen (protein involved in blood clotting) and other proteins leaking out of the capillary. The local inflammatory reaction to a soft tissue injury also includes an increase in both tissue metabolism and temperature.

The first step is the application of a **cold** pack to the injured area. Many people think that a cold pack has primarily an analgesic function because cold does in fact lead to temporary loss of feeling in the local area; it is thought that cold impulses bombard and override the pain receptors. In addition, cold causes vasoconstriction and decreases tissue metabolism. Vasoconstriction occurs to conserve heat. Constriction at the arteriolar end of the capillary bed reduces capillary filtration (refer to Figure 8-1). The reduction of the metabolic rate can be explained chemically. A 10° decrease in temperature will reduce the rate of chemical reactions by one half. Soft tissue injuries such as sprains or dislocations may result in torn muscles or ligaments, damaged nerves and blood vessels, hemorrhage, edema, and muscle spasm. Cold application is necessary to reduce the metabolic demands of the tissue, restrict hemorrhage, and prevent edema. The treatment of cold to an

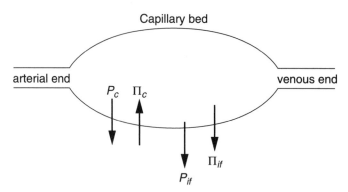

Figure 8-1 Illustration of a capillary bed and the Starling forces responsible for fluid flow across a capillary membrane.

injured area should be only 10–15 minutes per half hour to enable the tissue to receive nutrition.

Mobilization of the involved part is beneficial because muscle contraction and movement of the limb within the individual's pain-free range of motion are effective in removing excess fluid, improving the nutritional status of the tissue, and preventing soft tissue tightness and adhesions. Wrapping compresses the injured area and increases the interstitial fluid pressure, facilitating the movement of solutes and water from the interstitium into the lymphatic system.

The lymphatic system returns protein, water, and electrolytes from the interstitial spaces to the blood. If the lymphatic system has reached its maximum capability for fluid removal, edema will occur. The flow of lymph is dependent on the lymphatic pump and the fluid interstitial pressure. Compression of lymph vessels by muscle contraction, movement of body parts, arterial pulsations, and compression of the tissue by objects outside of the body will provide a pumping action which enhances lymph flow. Therefore, mobilization and compression are important for the movement of proteins and fluid into the lymphatic system.

The final part of the treatment is **elevation** of the injured area. Blood vessels may have been damaged as a result of injury. Elevation allows gravity to assist in returning the blood back to the heart. Elevation reduces the pressure at the venous end of the capillary bed which results in a decrease in capillary hydrostatic pressure (P_c).

We have established the function of mobilization, ice, compression and elevation in treating acute, soft tissue injuries. We can explain the effectiveness of MICE further by looking at fluid movement across the capillary wall as a result of hydrostatic or osmotic pressure differences. The Starling equation describes this relationship,

$$Jv = k\left[(P_c - P_{if}) - \sigma(\pi_c - \pi_{if})\right]$$

P_c = capillary fluid pressure k = filtration coefficient
P_{if} = interstitial fluid pressure σ = osmotic reflection coefficient
π_c = plasma colloid osmotic force   for plasma proteins
π_{if} = interstitial colloid osmotic force J_v = flow

The parameters of the Starling equation are illustrated in Figure 8-1. The filtration coefficient (k) of capillaries is proportional to the product of the capillary permeability to water and the surface area. The coefficient can be increased by opening capillary beds, thereby increasing the surface area. The value of the osmotic reflection coefficient for plasma proteins (σ) will range between zero and one. Zero represents that the membrane is freely permeable to proteins, and one represents total impermeability to protein. The pressure within the capillary (P_c) forces fluid out of the capillary. The fluid pressure in the interstitium (P_{if}) is negative under normal conditions and therefore pulls fluid out of the capillary. Plasma colloid osmotic force (π_c) develops in the capillary due to the presence of proteins; the colloid osmotic or oncotic pressure pulls fluid into the capillary. The interstitium also has a colloid osmotic force (π_{if}) which pulls fluid out of the capillary.

The forces counteract one another; under normal conditions, there is a small net flow of fluid out of the capillary. However, if large amounts of fluid leak out of the capillary in excess of the rate at which lymph can carry the fluid back to the blood, edema forms. The rate of lymph flow can be increased by any form of compression (previously mentioned) and factors which would increase interstitial fluid pressure (P_{if}). These factors include increasing capillary pressure (P_c), decreasing plasma colloid osmotic force (π_c), increasing protein in the interstitial fluid (π_{if}), and increasing the permeability of the capillaries. The following exercise was developed for students to further understand the relationship between the different forces responsible for fluid flow across the capillary membrane.

Materials

calculator, pencil, paper

Student Objectives

1. To understand the physiological basis of treating an injury such as a sprain with **M**obilization, **I**ce, **C**ompression, and **E**levation.
2. To be able to describe the forces responsible for filtration across the capillary membrane with Starling's equation.
3. To describe the changes in Starling forces as a result of **MICE** treatment.

STEP 1:   EXPERIMENTAL PROCEDURE

This exercise is designed to determine the effects of the standard treatment for a soft tissue injury (mobilization, ice, compression, and elevation) on the components of the Starling equation. Describe the changes in Starling forces (increase/decrease/no change) that you would expect to occur during the following situations and record them in Table 8-1:

A. Application of **COLD** to reduce blood flow to the area, prevent edema, and reduce the metabolic demands of the tissue.
B. **MOBILIZATION** within the individual's pain-free range of motion and **COMPRESSION** of the area with an ace bandage. Wrapping the injured area with an ace bandage or some other wrap applies **pressure** to the lymph vessels and, as with **mobilization,** facilitates the movement of lymph.
C. **ELEVATION** of the involved area increases blood flow back to the heart and lowers the pressure at the venous end of the capillary bed.

Table 8-1 Changes in the parameters of the Starling equation with MICE treatment (increase, decrease, or no change).

Treatment	P_{if}	P_c	π_{if}	π_c	k
Cold					
Mobilization					
Compression					
Elevation					

Discussion Questions

1. Explain the hydrostatic and osmotic forces responsible for fluid flow across the capillary membrane. Draw a picture representing the forces which cause flow in and out of the capillary. Why can P_{if} be considered a force which causes flow out of the capillary?
2. If the net movement of fluid is out of the capillary, why doesn't edema form?
3. The normal value of the filtration coefficient in the skeletal muscle bed is .007 ml/kg/mmHg/100 gm. During exercise, $k = .07$. What determines k and why would it increase during exercise?
4. Explain the use of compression and mobilization in terms of $\mathbf{P_{if}}$.

Answers to Exercise 8

A. The application of cold produces vasoconstriction; therefore, less blood reaches the capillary and capillary hydrostatic pressure, P_c, decreases. In addition, the filtration coefficient, k decreases because vasoconstriction reduces the surface area of the capillary, and cold reduces capillary permeability.
B. Initially, mobilization and compression increase the interstitial hydrostatic pressure, P_{if}, and increase the rate of lymph flow. Eventually, the fluid in the interstitium decreases. As a result interstitial hydrostatic pressure will decreases as well.

⇒ Point of Interest

Gentle massage of the area also facilitates the rate of lymph flow. Massage acts as an external pressure which will increase the interstitial hydrostatic pressure, P_{if} and increase lymph flow.

C. Elevation decreases the capillary hydrostatic pressure, P_c, because efferent arteriole pressure decreases and gravity assists in pulling blood toward the heart. Reduced pressure in the capillary ensures that less fluid will leak into the interstitium and increase P_{if}.

Answers to Discussion Questions

1. Picture should look like picture on page 80. P_{if} can be considered a force causing flow out of the capillary because it is negative under resting conditions.

2. The excess fluid is carried away by the lymph vessels. Under healthy, resting conditions the fluid leaking out of the capillaries is a small volume which can be handled by the lymphatic system.

3. The filtration coefficient, k, is determined by the capillary surface area and the capillary permeability to water. During exercise, more capillary beds open up to supply the active muscle with oxygen and nutrients, increasing the surface area and therefore increasing k.

4. Both compression and mobilization increase P_{if}. We do not want to maintain an increased interstitial hydrostatic pressure; however, it is a stimulus to increase the rate of lymph flow. Compression and mobilization apply pressure directly on the lymph vessels themselves and increase the rate of lymph flow. The lymph vessels carry the excess fluid away from the injured area and decrease the interstitial hydrostatic pressure. Edema can form if the lymphatic system has reached its capacity.

PART V Clinical Applications: Therapeutic Exercise

LABORATORY EXERCISE 9:   INTEGRATING CARDIOVASCULAR PRINCIPLES WITH PHYSICAL THERAPY MODALITIES

BACKGROUND AND THEORY

To evaluate an individual's aerobic capacity or cardiovascular fitness, the maximum oxygen uptake, $\dot{V}O_{2max}$, is measured. $\dot{V}O_{2max}$ is measured to assess the ability of the muscles to extract oxygen from the blood and the heart's ability to effectively pump blood to the active muscles. The Fick equation describes this relationship, $\dot{V}O_2 = CO \times (a - vO_2)$, where CO is the cardiac output and $(a - vO_2)$ is the difference in oxygen content between arterial and venous blood. Cardiac output is a function of heart rate and stroke volume ($HR \times SV = CO$). Therefore, maximum oxygen consumption is limited by the ability of the circulatory system to deliver oxygen and the ability of the muscle cells to utilize oxygen. The maximum oxygen uptake can be determined by performing a maximal exercise test, in which the individual exercises to exhaustion. However, performing at a maximal workload may be harmful to an individual, particularly if he or she is injured, recovering from surgery, or suffering from heart disease, insulin-dependent diabetes, or other pathological condition which reduces oxygen delivery to the tissues. Individuals with limiting conditions such as these may have their aerobic capacity evaluated by a method of **estimating** $\dot{V}O_{2max}$. To estimate $\dot{V}O_{2max}$, the subject exercises at a submaximal rate and the $\dot{V}O_{2max}$ is determined based on a steady state heart rate measurement obtained during the exercise bout. The exact steps to estimate maximum oxygen uptake are explained in the procedure section of this laboratory exercise.

[(SIt is essential to know the relationship between three parameters—**heart rate, work rate,** and **oxygen consumption**—in order to understand how the estimation of $\dot{V}O_{2max}$ is effective. There is a linear relationship between heart rate and oxygen uptake (Figure 9-1). Likewise, there is a linear relationship between work rate and heart rate. Therefore, we can demonstrate a linear relationship between oxygen uptake and work rate. The relationships among heart rate, work rate, and oxygen consumption are the basis for estimating $\dot{V}O_{2max}$. Exercise training alters the relationship between heart rate and oxygen consumption. Heart rate will still rise as $\dot{V}O_2$ increases; however, training allows an individual to provide the same amount of oxygen, but at a lower heart rate. Active skeletal muscle requires more oxygen and energy substrates (glucose, fat) to function. The nutrients are carried to the tissue by the blood. Because the demand for these nutrients is high during exercise, the heart must pump more blood to the tissue. The amount of blood pumped to the tissue per minute is the **cardiac output** (CO). CO is the product of **heart rate** (HR)

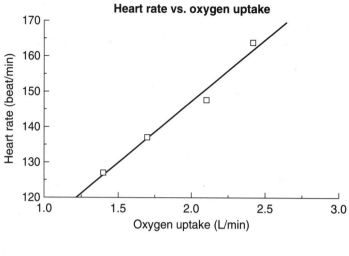

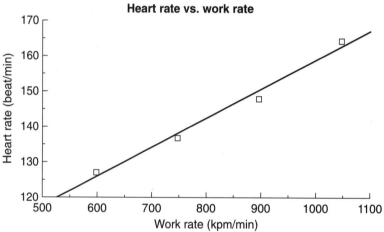

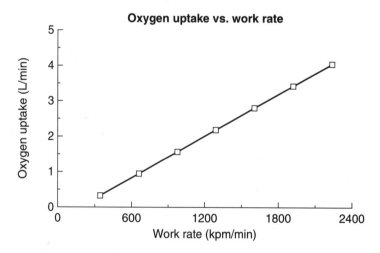

Figure 9-1   Relationship among heart rate, oxygen consumption, and workload.

and **stroke volume** (*SV*). With the onset of exercise, parasympathetic withdrawal and sympathetic discharge increase heart rate and contractility of the heart. The heart is able to eject more blood per beat, i.e., the stroke volume increases. Therefore, *CO* increases during exercise because both *HR* and *SV* increase. With training, an individual will achieve the same cardiac output as an untrained individual but at a lower heart rate due to the trained individual's greater stroke volume (Figure 9-2).

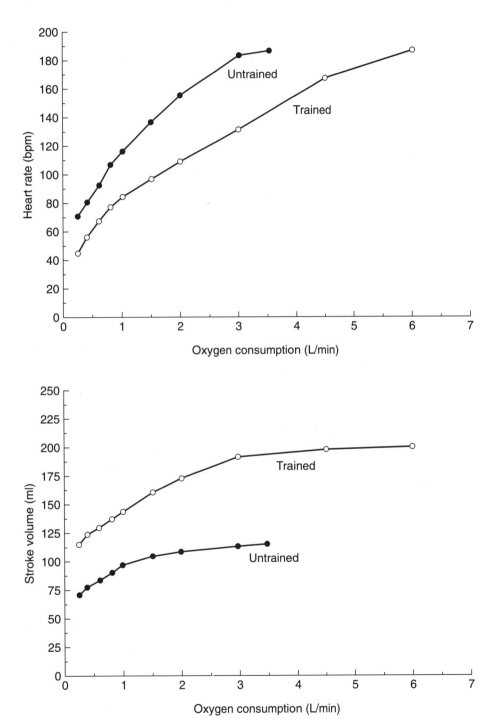

Figure 9-2 Relationship between heart rate, stroke volume, and workload in trained and untrained individuals.

Two variables, heart rate and work rate, are determined during the submaximal exercise test and used to estimate the third variable, oxygen uptake. From the heart rate versus oxygen uptake graph in Figure 9-3, prediction of $\dot{V}O_{2max}$ can be demonstrated as follows. First determine the subject's maximum heart rate. The rule of thumb is maximum heart rate = 220 − age in years. Draw a line from the point on the Y-axis representing maximum heart rate to the straight line of the graph. Drop a perpendicular line from that point down to the X-axis. The point where the perpendicular intersects the X-axis represents his or her $\dot{V}O_{2max}$.

$\dot{V}O_{2max}$ estimation is necessary to assess an individual's cardiovascular system and assist in planning an exercise program for that individual. Additionally, an individual's progress can be tracked by measuring (or estimating) $\dot{V}O_{2max}$ because maximum oxygen consumption increases with training. A less obvious function of determining one's $\dot{V}O_{2max}$ is to assure that an individual receives appropriate care/therapy in the clinic. For example, trained individuals cannot tolerate upright tilt as long as untrained individuals; the reflex responses to orthostatic stress are diminished in trained individuals. Recognizing an individual's $\dot{V}O_{2max}$ would allow you to predict how he or she would respond on the electronic tilt table. However, keep in mind that there is a genetic component of one's $\dot{V}O_{2max}$. An individual may

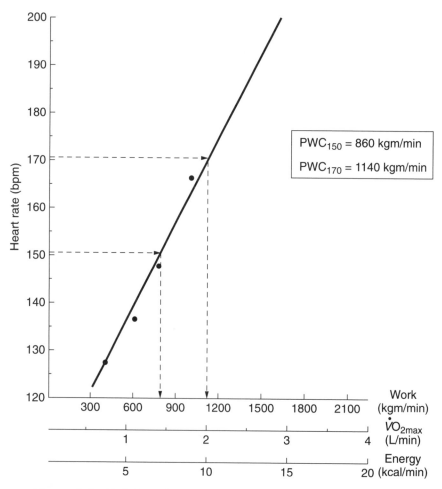

Figure 9-3 Relationship among work, oxygen consumption, and energy expenditure. (Physical work capacity determined at heart rates 150 and 170 bpm.)

have a high $\dot{V}O_{2max}$, comparable to the averages for a trained individual, yet the individual may not exercise regularly. You may also use an individual's $\dot{V}O_{2max}$ in order to develop an appropriate exercise program for him or her. If the individual is diabetic, he or she will respond better to shorter, more intense exercise bouts than a longer aerobic exercise bout. These are two examples, among many, illustrating the usefulness of the method of estimating $\dot{V}O_{2max}$.

With the addition of a few more steps we can also perform the **physical work capacity test** (PWC), another method of assessing an individual's level of fitness. The physical work capacity test takes advantage of the same relationships among heart rate, work rate, and oxygen uptake described previously (Figure 9-1). The exercise bout performed by the subject is submaximal; however, the work load is increased until the subject reaches a target heart rate. Heart rates ($>$120 bpm) taken during the exercise bouts are plotted on a graph of heart rate vs work rate, oxygen uptake and energy expenditure (Figure 9-3). The PWC_{170}, or, for older individuals the PWC_{140}, is the result of the test; it represents the work load required at a given heart rate. The subscript number is the individual's target heart rate. Target heart rate can be calculated by either method explained below in the sample calculations.

Sample 1:   resting heart rate = 60 bpm   age = 20 years

maximum heart rate = 220 − age = 200 bpm

max heart rate − resting heart rate = heart rate reserve

200 − 60 = 140 bpm

exercise within 60–80% heart rate reserve

140 × .6 = 84 bpm   140 × .8 = 112 bpm

60 + 84 = 144 bpm   60 + 112 = 172 bpm

The exercise subject should maintain a heart rate between 144 and 172 beats per minute throughout.

Sample 2:   maximum heart rate = 220 − age

200 = 220 − 20

70–80% maximum heart rate represents 60–80% heart rate reserve

200 × .7 = 140 bpm   200 × .8 = 160 bpm

The range of target heart rates is similar to that determined in Sample 1.

The maximum oxygen uptake test ($\dot{V}O_{2max}$) indicates the maximal work capacity, however, the PWC test provides information about the subject's response to increasing intensities of exercise. The PWC is a useful tool for determining the activities an individual could perform if he or she were limited to activities during which his or her heart rate could not exceed a given value. If an individual had diabetes and required hospitalization, a PWC test would be necessary to help the physician maintain the patient's blood glucose levels. Exercise functions as insulin (increasing the utilization of glucose); therefore, a patient admitted to the hospital will need to perform daily exercises equivalent in caloric expenditure to that of his or her daily activities in order to maintain his or her glucose levels. The PWC is also the basis for exercise prescription; the appropriate exercise intensity can be determined based on the individual's response to the graded exercise bout.

The cycle ergometer will be used to perform the submaximal exercise test and the physical work capacity test. The mechanical efficiency of cycle riding is nearly the same for all riders of varying skill and is independent of body weight, within limits. Therefore, each student consumes the same amount of oxygen when cycling at a given work rate.

Materials

cycle ergometer, tilt table
metronome, scale
sphygmomanometer, stethoscope

Student Objectives

1. To learn how to estimate an individual's maximum oxygen uptake and perform the physical work capacity (PWC) test to determine an individual's level of fitness.
2. To learn how to utilize $\dot{V}O_{2max}$ as a tool.
3. To observe the effects of using a common therapeutic device (tilt table) and understand the physiology of upright tilt.
4. To compare anaerobic and aerobic capacities among students in the class.
5. To understand the cardiovascular response to training.
6. To utilize the relationships among heart rate, work rate, oxygen uptake, and energy expenditure to prescribe exercise for a patient with heart disease and an individual with diabetes.

STEP 1: ESTIMATING MAXIMUM OXYGEN CONSUMPTION AND PERFORMING THE PHYSICAL WORK CAPACITY TEST

Cycle Ergometer

This laboratory exercise was designed to introduce the student to the effects of exercise, particularly on the cardiovascular system. Students will also realize the importance of determining one's level of fitness before treatment.

1. The subject should be dressed in gym clothes and have refrained from caffeine, eating, and smoking at least two hours prior to the test.
2. Record the weight of the subject in kilograms while dressed, but without his or her shoes. Enter the weight and age of the subject on Table 9-1.
3. Adjust the seat and set the resistance indicator of the cycle ergometer to zero. The subject's knee should be nearly extended with the foot pedal in the down position. Failure to extend the knee completely while pedaling may lead to premature fatigue in the leg and impaired venous return.

Table 9-1 Data necessary to calculate $\dot{V}O_{2max}$ (including age, weight) and a table for recording heart rate during the last 30 seconds of each minute of the submaximal exercise test.

Weight (kg) = _____

Age (years) = _____

Heart rate (beat/min)

Trials	1	2	3	4	5	6
Work rate (kgm)						
Time (min)						
1						
2						
3						
4						
5						
6						
Average HR of 5th & 6th min						

Estimated $\dot{V}O_{2max}$ (L/min) = _____

Age corrected $\dot{V}O_{2max}$ (L/min) = _____

Relative $\dot{V}O_{2max}$ (ml/kg/min) = _____

METS (1 MET = 3.5 ml/kg/min) = _____

Level of fitness (circle one)   LOW   AVERAGE   HIGH

4. The subject should begin pedaling the cycle ergometer at 50 pedal-revolutions per minute. The rate of 50 rpm was chosen because it has been determined that between 50 rpm and 60 rpm, the greatest efficiency of cycle riding is obtained by an individual regardless of weight or size. The work load should then be set at 1 kg (300 kgm/min) for women and 2 kg (600 kgm/min) for men. Continue the exercise bout for six minutes. Record the work load on Table 9-1.

5. Record heart rate during the last 30 seconds of every minute of exercise in column 1 of Table 9-1. See the appendix for instructions on how to obtain accurate heart rate measurements. The average heart rate from the fifth and sixth minutes of exercise will be used to estimate the maximum oxygen uptake. If the work load does not produce a heart rate greater than 120 beats per minute, increase the work load by 150 kgm and repeat the six-minute exercise bout. At heart rates less than 120, the linear relationship between heart rate and oxygen consumption does not exist because at heart rates below 120, heart rate and stroke volume increase. Beyond 170 bpm, the oxygen consumption is no longer linearly related with heart rate because the $(a-v\ O_2)$ starts to increase.

6. To complete the physical work capacity test, allow the subject to rest for five minutes. Increase the work load by 150 kgm and repeat the six-minute exercise bout, recording heart rate during the last 30 seconds of each minute. Repeat six-minute exercise bouts at increasing work loads until the individual's target heart rate is reached or at least three heart rates greater than 120 bpm have been recorded. Allow the subject to rest five minutes between each six-minute bout. Remember to record heart rate and the corresponding work load in Table 9-1.

7. Determine the estimated $\dot{V}O_{2max}$ according to Table 9-2a (or b). You need the mean heart rate for the fifth and sixth minutes and the work rate at which the heart rate was attained from the first trial (column 1, Table 9-1).

8. Age is the major factor in determining maximum heart rate. Because heart rate and $\dot{V}O_{2max}$ are linearly related, $\dot{V}O_{2max}$ must be corrected for age. Consult the age correction table, Table 9-3, and adjust the value for the subject's age by multiplying the $\dot{V}O_{2max}$ value by the correction factor.

9. Determine the relative $\dot{V}O_{2max}$. Divide the $\dot{V}O_{2max}$ calculated in step 7 by the subject's weight in kilograms. Convert the value to milliliters per kilogram per minute (ml/kg/min).

10. Convert $\dot{V}O_{2max}$ (ml/kg/min) to **metabolic equivalents** (METS). One MET is the average oxygen cost at rest per kilogram body weight, or 3.5 ml/kg/min.

11. Consult Table 9-4 to categorize your level of aerobic fitness based on the estimated relative $\dot{V}O_{2max}$.

12. The PWC_{150} and PWC_{170} will be determined by the values recorded in Table 9-1 and completion of the graph in Figure 9-4. Plot heart rate values (≥ 120) obtained during the increasing work loads on the graph. Draw a line of best fit between the points such that an equal number of points will lie on either side of the line.

13. Draw a horizontal line from the Y-axis at 170 beat/min to the line of best fit. From that point, draw a perpendicular line down to the X-axis. The intersection of the line and the X-axis represents the PWC_{170}. The same procedure should be done to determine the PWC_{150}.

STEP 2: RESPONSE TO UPRIGHT TILT

Methods for Studying the Response to Upright Tilt

1. Estimate the aerobic capacity by use of the submaximal exercise test on a cycle ergometer for each subject.

2. Average maximum oxygen uptake values and categorize subjects into above average fit and below average fit groups. Record mean $\dot{V}O_{2max}$ values on Table 9-5. The average height and weight for each group should also be recorded. Proceed with the tilt test described next.

3. Each subject should rest supine on the electronic tilt table for 30 minutes.

4. Record blood pressure every five minutes on Table 9-6; monitor ECG and heart rate responses.

5. Raise the tilt table to 70° head up tilt. Record blood pressure and heart rate after each minute for five minutes on Table 9-6.

Table 9-2a Predicted maximum oxygen uptake for men based on work rate and corresponding heart rate.

Heart Rate	300 kpm/min	600 kpm/min	900 kpm/min	1200 kpm/min	1500 kpm/min
120	2.2	3.5	4.8		
121	2.2	3.4	4.7		
122	2.2	3.4	4.6		
123	2.1	3.4	4.6		
124	2.1	3.3	4.5	6.0	
125	2.0	3.2	4.4	5.9	
126	2.0	3.2	4.4	5.8	
127	2.0	3.1	4.3	5.7	
128	2.0	3.1	4.2	5.6	
129	1.9	3.0	4.2	5.6	
130	1.9	3.0	4.1	5.5	
131	1.9	2.9	4.0	5.4	
132	1.8	2.9	4.0	5.3	
133	1.8	2.8	3.9	5.3	
134	1.8	2.8	3.9	5.2	
135	1.7	2.8	3.8	5.1	
136	1.7	2.7	3.8	5.0	
137	1.7	2.7	3.7	5.0	
138	1.6	2.7	3.7	4.9	
139	1.6	2.6	3.6	4.8	
140	1.6	2.6	3.6	4.8	6.0
141		2.6	3.5	4.7	5.9
142		2.5	3.5	4.6	5.8
143		2.5	3.4	4.6	5.7
144		2.5	3.4	4.5	5.7
145		2.4	3.4	4.5	5.6
146		2.4	3.3	4.4	5.6

Heart Rate	300 kpm/min	600 kpm/min	900 kpm/min	1200 kpm/min	1500 kpm/min
147		2.4		4.4	5.5
148		2.4		4.3	5.4
149		2.3		4.3	5.4
150		2.3		4.2	5.3
151		2.3		4.2	5.2
152		2.3		4.1	5.2
153		2.2		4.1	5.1
154		2.2		4.0	5.1
155		2.2		4.0	5.0
156		2.2		4.0	5.0
157		2.1		3.9	4.9
158		2.1		3.9	4.9
159		2.1		3.8	4.8
160		2.1		3.8	4.8
161		2.0		3.7	4.7
162		2.0		3.7	4.6
163		2.0		3.7	4.6
164		2.0		3.6	4.5
165		2.0		3.6	4.5
166		1.9		3.6	4.5
167		1.9		3.5	4.4
168		1.9		3.5	4.4
169		1.9		3.5	4.3
170		1.8		3.4	4.3

Table 9-2b Predicted maximum oxygen uptake for women based on work rate and corresponding heart rate.

Heart Rate	300 kpm/min	450 kpm/min	600 kpm/min	750 kpm/min	900 kpm/min
120	2.6	3.4	4.1	4.8	
121	2.5	3.3	4.0	4.8	
122	2.5	3.2	3.9	4.7	
123	2.4	3.1	3.9	4.6	
124	2.4	3.1	3.8	4.5	
125	2.3	3.0	3.7	4.4	
126	2.3	3.0	3.6	4.3	
127	2.2	2.9	3.5	4.2	
128	2.2	2.8	3.5	4.2	4.8
129	2.2	2.8	3.4	4.1	4.8
130	2.1	2.7	3.4	4.0	4.7
131	2.1	2.7	3.4	4.0	4.6
132	2.0	2.7	3.3	3.9	4.5
133	2.0	2.6	3.2	3.8	4.4
134	2.0	2.6	3.2	3.8	4.4
135	2.0	2.6	3.1	3.7	4.3
136	1.9	2.5	3.1	3.6	4.2
137	1.9	2.5	3.0	3.6	4.2
138	1.8	2.4	3.0	3.5	4.1
139	1.8	2.4	2.9	3.5	4.0
140	1.8	2.4	2.8	3.4	4.0
141	1.8	2.3	2.8	3.4	3.9
142	1.7	2.3	2.8	3.3	3.9
143	1.7	2.2	2.7	3.3	3.8
144	1.7	2.2	2.7	3.2	3.8
145	1.6	2.2	2.7	3.2	3.7
146	1.6	2.2	2.6	3.2	3.7

Heart Rate	300 kpm/min	450 kpm/min	600 kpm/min	750 kpm/min	900 kpm/min
147	1.6	2.1	2.6	3.1	3.6
148	1.6	2.1	2.6	3.1	3.6
149		2.1	2.6	3.0	3.5
150		2.0	2.5	3.0	3.5
151		2.0	2.5	3.0	3.4
152		2.0	2.5	2.9	3.4
153		2.0	2.4	2.9	3.3
154		2.0	2.4	2.8	3.3
155		1.9	2.4	2.8	3.2
156		1.9	2.3	2.8	3.2
157		1.9	2.3	2.7	3.2
158		1.8	2.3	2.7	3.1
159		1.8	2.2	2.7	3.1
160		1.8	2.2	2.6	3.0
161		1.8	2.2	2.6	3.0
162		1.8	2.2	2.6	3.0
163		1.7	2.2	2.6	2.9
164		1.7	2.1	2.5	2.9
165		1.7	2.1	2.5	2.9
166		1.7	2.1	2.5	2.8
167		1.6	2.1	2.4	2.8
168		1.6	2.0	2.4	2.8
169		1.6	2.0	2.4	2.8
170		1.6	2.0	2.4	2.7

Table 9-3   Age correction factors.*

Age	Factor
15	1.1
25	1.00
35	.87
40	.83
50	.75

*Correction factor is .01 per year between ages 15–25.

Table 9-4   Fitness classification for men and women based on maximal oxygen uptake. Values represent relative $\dot{V}O_{2max}$ (ml/kg/min).

Age	Low	Average	High
Women			
20–29	32	33–43	44
30–39	31	32–41	42
40–49	29	30–40	41
Men			
20–29	41	42–51	52
30–39	37	38–47	48
40–49	33	34–43	44

**Tables 9-2, 9-3, and 9-4 are adapted from Astrand, P. O., *Ergometry—Test of "Physical Fitness,"* Varberg, Sweden: Monark Crescent AB, as adapted from Astrand, I., "Aerobic work capacity in men and women with special reference to age," *Acta Physiol. Scand.,* 49 (suppl. 169): 45–60, 83, 1960.

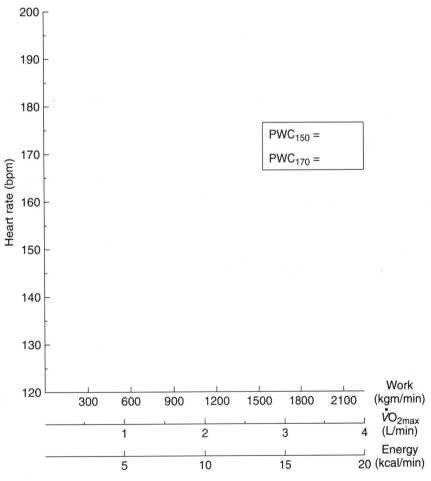

Figure 9-4   Plot heart rate at each work load to determine the PWC at 150 and 170 bpm.

Table 9-5 Group Demographic Data.

Characteristics	Above average group	Below average group
Age		
Height		
Weight		
Maximum MET*		

*One metabolic equivalent (MET) equals the average oxygen cost at rest per kilogram body weight, or 3.5ml/kg/min.

Table 9-6 Hemodynamic responses of above average (AA) and below average (BA) groups to upright tilt.

	Tilt (minutes)				
	Control	1	2	3	4
Heart Rate (beat/min)					
BA					
AA					
Systolic blood pressure (mmHg)					
BA					
AA					
Diastolic blood pressure (mmHg)					
BA					
AA					
Mean arterial pressure (mmHg)					
BA					
AA					
Pulse pressure (mmHg)					
BA					
AA					

6. Return tilt table to horizontal plane. Allow the subject to recover for 15 minutes.

7. Plot the average values for the hemodynamic parameters from Table 9-6 on Figures 9-5 to 9-10.

8. It has already been mentioned that trained and untrained individuals respond differently to orthostatic stress. The neural reflex responsible for maintaining arterial blood pressure may be less sensitive and therefore not respond as quickly to a fall in blood pressure in the trained individual. This mechanism is the **baroreceptor reflex** (Figure 9-11). Baroreceptors, located in the carotid sinus and aortic arch, send afferent signals to the nucleus tractus solitaris (NTS) of the brainstem when arterial blood pressure increases. These signals inhibit the sympathetic (vasoconstrictor) center and activate the vagal center of the brain. Vagal efferents are sent to the heart to slow the heart rate. When an individual stands after having been lying down, there is an immediate decrease in arterial blood pressure. Upon standing, there is a redistribution of blood, such that blood pools in the extremities due to the force of gravity. As blood pools in the peripheral vessels, there is a temporary decrease in venous return and therefore stroke volume. Stroke volume is a determinant of arterial blood pressure; therefore, a decrease in stroke volume contributes to a decrease in arterial blood pressure. In this situation, less afferent signals travel to the NTS due to the pressure drop. The result is the withdrawal of vagal activity and increased discharge of sympathetic activity. The sympathetic efferent nerves will travel to the heart and vasculature to increase contractility and vasoconstrict, respectively. Withdrawal of vagal tone will result in an increase in heart rate. It is comparable to letting your foot off the break of your

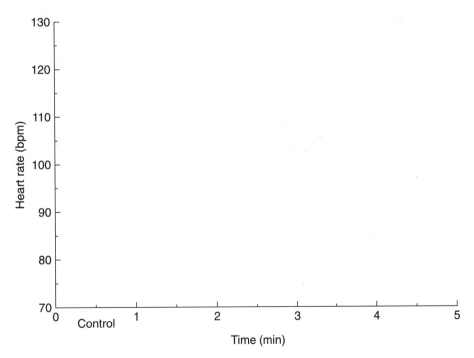

Figure 9-5   Heart rate at rest and during each minute of upright tilt.

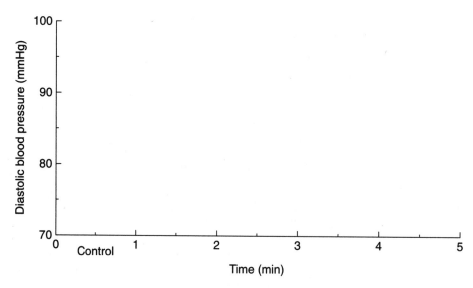

Figure 9-6   Diastolic blood pressure response at rest and during upright tilt.

car, i.e., the car speeds up. Mean arterial pressure (*MAP*) is the product of cardiac output (*CO*) and total peripheral resistance (*TPR*), $MAP = CO \times TPR$.

By increasing the heart rate, *CO* increases and *MAP* increases. Likewise, vasoconstriction (enhanced sympathetic activity) increases vascular resistance and therefore increases *MAP*. Heart rate and the degree of vasomotor tone are determined by the amount of sympathetic and vagal input. The baroreceptor reflex functions to maintain arterial blood pressure relatively constant by turning on/off sympathetic/vagal centers in the brain. Determine baroreceptor sensitivity for the above and below average groups by calculating **gain.**

Gain = Change in *HR*/change in pulse pressure

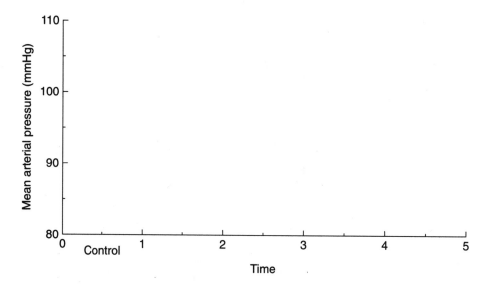

Figure 9-7   Mean arterial pressure at rest and during upright tilt.

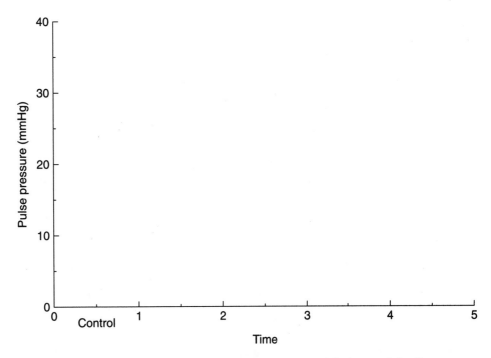

Figure 9-8   Pulse pressure response at rest and during upright tilt.

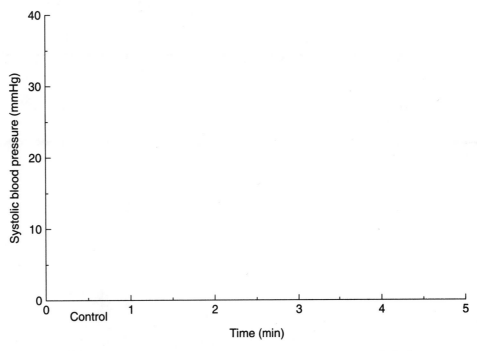

Figure 9-9   Systolic blood pressure response at rest and during upright tilt.

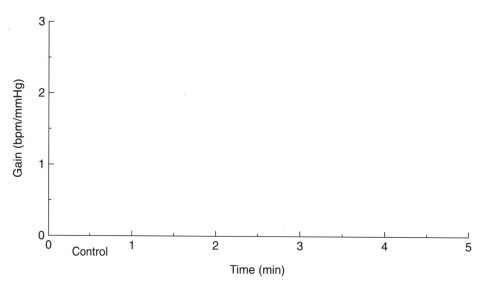

Figure 9-10 Baroreceptor sensitivity calculated as change rate/change in pulse pressure.

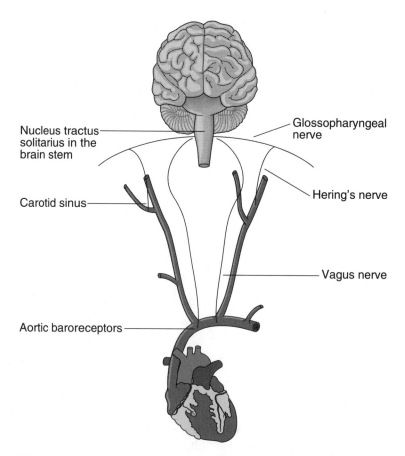

Figure 9-11 This figure illustrates the afferent signals of the baroreceptor reflex. A pressure change in the aortic arch is sensed by the aortic baroreceptors which send signals to the NTS through the vagus nerve. The carotid sinus baroreceptors send signals to the NTS through Hering's nerve and the glossopharyngeal nerve.

9. Construct a bar graph representing the average gain for the below average and above average groups on Figure 9-11.

Discussion Questions

1. What was your estimated $\dot{V}O_{2max}$? How does it compare with the average $\dot{V}O_{2max}$ values of the students in your class?
2. Describe the changes in heart rate and blood pressure (pulse pressure, systolic pressure, diastolic pressure, mean arterial pressure) that occurred in response to upright tilt.
3. Compare the hemodynamic parameters between the above average and below average fit groups.
4. Which group would you expect to have a higher average gain? Did this occur?

STEP 3:   AEROBIC vs ANAEROBIC CAPACITY

Based on theory and clinical practice, students might expect to find gender influences on aerobic and anaerobic capacity. Therefore, the objective in the second part of this laboratory exercise is to determine if there is a gender difference in aerobic and anaerobic capacities. **Aerobic capacity** refers to an individual's ability to perform exercise bouts which require oxygen to provide the energy source to maintain that activity. It is a function of the respiratory, cardiovascular, and metabolic systems working to maximize the oxygen consumption, transport, and utilization. **Anaerobic capacity** is the individual's ability to sustain high-intensity exercise bouts in which the body utilizes the breakdown of stored ATP and creatine phosphate to provide energy for the first 30 seconds of an exercise bout. The breakdown of muscle glycogen (anaerobic glycolysis) is another source of energy (ATP) during anaerobic exercise bouts. An individual can maintain a high-intensity exercise bout for approximately four minutes utilizing the breakdown of muscle glycogen. The aerobic pathways of energy utilization are too slow to provide the substrates to maintain this type of exercise bout. Anaerobic exercise bouts are of short duration because the energy stores are rapidly depleted. Conversely, aerobic exercise bouts are of longer duration and lower intensity. Each student will be required to participate in an exercise bout at 60% of the estimated $\dot{V}O_{2max}$ which will represent an aerobic exercise bout, and a second exercise bout at 90% of the estimated $\dot{V}O_{2max}$, which will represent an anaerobic exercise bout. The exercise bouts will continue until fatigue. Fatigue will be indicated when the subject can no longer maintain the specified (50 rpm) rate of pedaling the cycle ergometer. Patients with diabetes actually respond better to anaerobic exercise than aerobic exercise. The time to fatigue at 90% of estimated $\dot{V}O_{2max}$ is longer in diabetic patients than in non-diabetic individuals, and the time to fatigue at 60% of the estimated $\dot{V}O_{2max}$ is shorter in diabetic individuals than in non-diabetic individuals. Individuals with diabetes have adapted to poor oxygen delivery to the tissues by enhancing their anaerobic capacity. The average time to fatigue for the male students will be calculated for the exercise bouts of both intensities. The average time to fatigue for the female students will be calculated for the exercise bouts of both intensities.

1. Divide the class into two groups, male students in one group and female students in the second group.

2. Calculate the average age, height, weight, and estimated $\dot{V}O_{2max}$ for male and female students if this has not already been done earlier. Complete Table 9-5.

3. Calculate the work rate required to have the subject achieve 60% or 90% of $\dot{V}O_{2max}$. Multiply the subject's $\dot{V}O_{2max}$ by 0.6 or 0.9. Locate this value on Figure 9-4 (Step 1) from the PWC test. From the relationship between oxygen uptake and work rate, the work rate required for a subject to perform can be estimated. From the point on the line of best fit corresponding to the percent $\dot{V}O_{2max}$, locate the corresponding point on the X-axis labeled **Work.** This point represents the work rate necessary for the subject to achieve 60 or 90% of $\dot{V}O_{2max}$.

4. Each student should complete two exercise bouts, the first at 60% of $\dot{V}O_{2max}$ to fatigue and the second at 90% of $\dot{V}O_{2max}$ to fatigue. The first exercise bout (60% of $\dot{V}O_{2max}$) is an aerobic exercise bout. The second exercise (90% of $\dot{V}O_{2max}$) represents an anaerobic exercise bout. The index of fatigue used in this exercise will be the point at which the subject can no longer maintain 50 rpm (±5).

   TIME TO FATIGUE AT 60% of $\dot{V}O_{2max}$_____

   TIME TO FATIGUE AT 90% of $\dot{V}O_{2max}$_____

5. Calculate the average time to fatigue for the male and female students at both intensities of exercise. Complete Table 9-7.

6. Construct a bar graph representing the average time to fatigue while exercising at 60% of $\dot{V}O_{2max}$ for male and female students in Figure 9-12.

7. Construct a bar graph representing the average time to fatigue while exercising at 90% of $\dot{V}O_{2max}$ for male and female students in Figure 9-13.

Discussion Questions

1. Was there a gender difference in the average time to fatigue with exercise bouts at 60% of $\dot{V}O_{2max}$?

2. Was there a gender difference in the average time to fatigue with exercise bouts at 90% of $\dot{V}O_{2max}$?

3. In response to questions 1 and 2, if differences were found between the male and female groups, suggest possible reasons for this.

Table 9-7   Average time to fatigue for male and female students at 60% of $\dot{V}O_{2max}$ and 90% of $\dot{V}O_{2max}$.

Intensity (%)	Male (n =)	Female (n =)
60		
90		

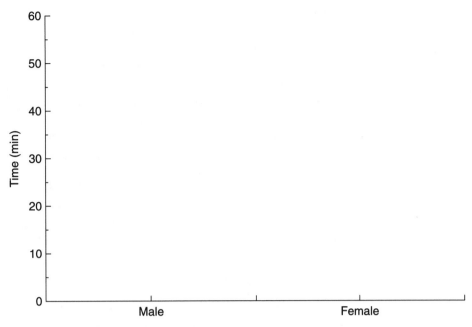

Figure 9-12   Time to fatigue during aerobic exercise bout (60% of $\dot{V}O_{2max}$).

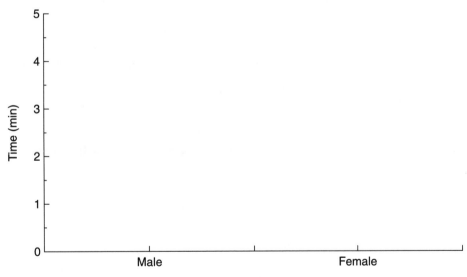

Figure 9-13   Time to fatigue during anaerobic exercise bout (90% of $\dot{V}O_{2max}$).

STEP 4:   TWO CASE STUDIES

Case Study 1

A male, age 57, was directed to the physical therapy clinic three weeks after having had balloon angioplasty to open right and left carotid arteries which were 50% and 80% blocked respectively. He came into the clinic feeling "great." He was an active sports enthusiast and was eager to begin working out again. Before surgery, he exercised at least four times per week. The following is a list of activities in which he participated before the surgery: playing basketball in a men's league one night a week, doubles tennis with his wife, jogging or walking 5 miles with his dog every other morning, swimming, and golfing. He owns his own landscaping business; while his sons perform most of the labor, he occasionally helps out on special projects or to meet the deadlines. The labor may involve shoveling stones or mulch, pushing full wheelbarrows, and lifting shrubs and trees in excess of 50 pounds.

His physician sent him to the clinic to have a physical work capacity test done after his EKG stress test showed no irregular heart patterns, but his heart rate should not exceed 150 bpm. You are to determine which activities he can participate in without risk. The results of the PWC_{150} test are listed below. Plot them on Figure 9-14 and determine the PWC_{150}. According to the list of activities and their MET value, prescribe an exercise program for him. Choose activities which are 40–80% his maximum MET value.

Results of PWC test.

Heart rate (beat/min)	Work load (kgm/min)
120	450
135	600
148	750
	900

Weight = 70 kg.

Guideline of values to calculate in order to complete exercise prescription:

PWC_{150} = _____ kgm/min

PWC_{150} corresponds to _____ L/min

and _____ kcal/min

$\dot{V}O_{2max}$ = _____ ml/kg/min

Max METS = _____

Activities that are safe to perform:

Case Study 2

A 12-year-old girl was admitted to the hospital to have tests run that span three days. She has diabetes mellitus (insulin dependent) and will require insulin injections daily. However, she will not be able to perform her daily activities while she is in the hospital. Exercise increases the glucose uptake by the muscle as does insulin. Her physician wants to know how much insulin she will need while in the hospital. The physician wants to know her average daily energy expenditure and have an exercise program designed for the patient while she is staying in the hospital.

A record of all the activities she participated in during the past three days (prior to entering the hospital) needs to be completed also. Each activity will be listed along with the energy cost (calories/min) of performing that activity. The sum total of the calories/day will be given to the physician. You need to design an exercise bout in which the patient will expend energy, equivalent to the sum on the three-day

Table 9-8 Activities in METS.

	Mean	Range
Badminton	5.8	4–9
Basketball—game	8.3	7–12
—non-game	—	3–9
Bicycling	—	3–8
Dancing (square, social)	—	3.7–7.4
Golfing—power cart	—	2–3
—walking	5.1	4–7
Running—		
—12 min. mile	8.7	
—9 min. mile	11.2	
—6 min. mile	16.3	
Skating (ice or roller)	—	5–8
Skiing—downhill	—	5–8
—cross country	—	6–12
Stairclimbing	—	4–6
Swimming	—	4–8
Tennis	6.5	4–9
Gardening	3.6 (weeding)	
	6.5 (digging)	
Heavy lifting	—	6.0–7.7
Wheelbarrow (45 kg load)	—	3–4
Shoveling (snow, dirt)	—	5.0–7.0
Volleyball	—	3.0–6.0

Abbreviated table from American College of Sports Medicine, *Guidelines for Exercise Testing and Prescription*, Philadelphia: Lea & Febiger, 1991, pp. 104–105.

activity profile; this activity (treadmill, cycle ergometer) will be performed each day that she is hospitalized as a replacement of her daily activities.

Average energy expenditure for three days prior to hospital stay is shown below. Exercise needs to be prescribed to replace the moderate and heavy activities that she performs daily.

Activity	Time (min)	kcal per day
Sleeping	420	462
Light	120	480
Moderate	60	480
Heavy	90	900

The physical work capacity test was performed. The results of the test are listed below. Plot the heart rate values on Figure 9-15 in order to determine her PWC_{170}.

Heart rate (beat/min)	Work load (kgm/min)
115	300
124	450
137	600
150	750
162	900

Weight = 80 lbs.

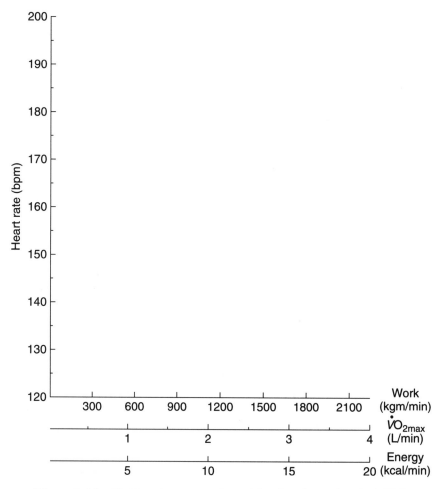

Figure 9-14   Plot heart rate at each work load to determine the PWC at 150 bpm.

Guidelines of values to calculate in order to complete exercise prescription:

PWC$_{150}$ = _____ kgm/min
PWC$_{150}$ corresponds to _____ L/min
                    and _____ kcal/min
$\dot{V}O_{2max}$ = _____ ml/kg/min
Max METS = _____

Activities that are safe to perform:

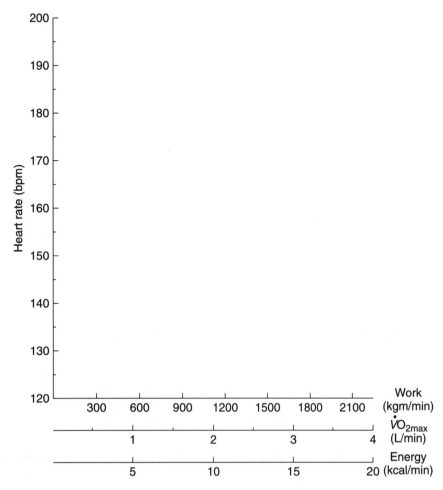

Figure 9-15   Plot heart rate at each work load to determine the PWC at 170 bpm.

Guidelines of values to calculate in order to complete exercise prescription:

PWC_{170} = _____ kgm/min
PWC_{170} corresponds to _____ L/min
                                    and _____ kcal/min
$\dot{V}O_{2max}$ = _____ ml/kg/min
Max METS = _____

Excercise should be at 600kgm and she must expend 1400 kcal.
Length of excercise bout _____ minutes

Appendix

OBTAINING HEART RATE MEASUREMENTS

To obtain heart rate measurements follow these steps. Using your fingers and not your thumb, feel the pulse on the radial (thumb side) portion of the student's wrist or on the neck at the carotid artery. Count the number of beats in 10 seconds. Multiply the number of beats by six to obtain a heart rate expressed as beats per minute. Be careful when obtaining heart rate from the carotid artery (neck). If you apply too much pressure on the carotid artery, reflex slowing of the heart rate will occur.

OBTAINING BLOOD PRESSURE MEASUREMENTS

To measure blood pressure with the sphygmomanometer or blood pressure cuff follow these steps. Blood pressure measurements will only be taken during step 2.

1. The subject should be sitting on the bike, but resting for five minutes before a resting measurement is obtained.
2. Firmly, place the blood pressure cuff around the arm at the level of the heart. Do not remove the cuff after taking the resting blood pressure because the cuff needs to be on the subject's arm during the entire experiment.
3. Locate the point that the brachial artery passes over the elbow. Palpate the **brachial pulse** on the medial side of the groove in the anterior surface of the elbow. Mark this point with a water soluble marker. You will place the stethoscope over this site when measuring blood pressure.
4. Inflate the pressure cuff to 180 mmHg for resting measurements of blood pressure. During exercise, inflate the cuff between 200 and 220 mmHg. After inflating the cuff, place the stethoscope over the point marked in step 3.
5. **Slowly** release the pressure. The pressure should fall 2 to 3 mmHg per second. Listen for sound changes.
6. Identify and record the systolic and diastolic pressures

Systolic pressure.   The pressure at which you can hear a soft, thumping sound following the "slow release" of pressure in step 5. The sound indicates blood flow. The heart has developed a great enough force during systole to force blood past the cuff.

Diastolic pressure.   The pressure at which the sound disappears following a gradual increase in the sound and a "loud tapping effect." As the pressure in the cuff is lowered, blood is still forced past the occlusion. The pressure in the artery at end diastole is great enough to force blood by the occluding cuff. Sound disappears when the cuff has no occluding effect on blood flow in the brachial artery.

LABORATORY EXERCISE 10: ANALYSIS AND COMPARISON OF RATE PRESSURE PRODUCT, METS, AND OXYGEN CONSUMPTION FOR EXERCISE PRESCRIPTION

BACKGROUND AND THEORY

Physical therapists prescribe exercise to most of their patients, particularly those recovering from surgery, cardiac infarction, or acute injury in order to assist the patient in a complete recovery. Calisthenics are prescribed primarily according to the energy cost or the oxygen requirement of performing such an activity, e.g., abduction of the arms to the horizontal position followed by a biceps curl costs 1.5 METS. The product of heart rate and blood pressure is the double product (DP) or rate pressure product (RPP). There have been several studies published which correlate the heart rate and blood pressure response (both elevated) to exercise with the myocardial oxygen consumption ($M\dot{V}O_2$), i.e., RPP is highly correlated with $M\dot{V}O_2$.

The heart and vasculature adapt to the conditions encountered during the performance of muscular exercise. The muscular activity may be isotonic or isometric, but most likely a combination of the two. Swimming, running, and bicycling are primarily isotonic activities, whereas weight lifting with heavy resistance is predominantly an isometric activity.

The cardiovascular responses to isotonic exercise include increases in cardiac output, heart rate, and stroke volume in order to meet the high oxygen demand ($\dot{V}O_2 = CO \times (a - vO_2)$ and $CO = HR \times SV$). Conversely, oxygen demands increase minimally with isometric contractions; however, mean arterial pressure and heart rate increase markedly. Isometric activities place a pressure load on the heart which increases the oxygen demand of the heart without increasing the systemic oxygen consumption.

There are numerous calisthenics with the same MET values; however, two different exercises requiring the same amount of energy may involve different muscle groups, and generate varying degrees of tachycardia (increase heart rate) and hypertension. Calisthenics involving the upper extremities generate a higher heart rate and blood pressure than a calisthenic of equal METS involving the lower extremities. Calisthenics which consist of dynamic arm movements contain a large isometric component, i.e., static contraction of the trunk and hips for stability. While any form of resistance training increases the work of the heart, researchers have shown that isometric contractions significantly increase blood pressure beyond that produced by isotonic or isokinetic contractions. The elevation of blood pressure is proportional to the percent of maximal voluntary contraction (%MVC) of the muscle, not the size or absolute force produced. In 1984, M. Greer showed that 75% of MVC was less demanding on the cardiovascular system than isometric contractions at 100% of MVC.[1] Greer also found that the increases in heart rate and blood pressure were less when brief periods of rest were introduced or when the speed of the exercise decreased. Similarly, DiCarlo and Leonardo changed the technique of a typical arm exercise and observed large changes in heart rate, blood pressure, and rate pressure product without changing METS.[2] Their experiment consisted of healthy participants performing four variations of an arm exercise; the variations were in the speed and continuity of performing the exercise. Coinciding with the work of Greer, they found that the introduction of a pause within the exercise significantly reduced the heart rate, blood pressure, and rate pressure product without changing the MET value.

The appropriateness of prescribing exercise based on METS is limited. Perhaps the rate pressure product produced by a given calisthenic is a better indicator of the level of intensity. Individuals frequenting the clinic often have pre-existing conditions which may put them at risk when performing a calisthenic with high static component. For example, individuals with diabetes, hypertension, or heart disease already have compromised cardiovascular systems. Those individuals should have exercises prescribed to them based on the load the calisthenic places on the heart. The rate pressure product can be used as a functional indicator of the individual's level of exercise, rather than METS, because it represents the cardiovascular adaptation to the exercise. The following exercise was designed to illustrate these concepts.

Materials

timers, metronome
sphygmomanometers, stethoscopes

Student Objectives

1. To practice obtaining accurate heart rate and blood pressure readings in exercising subjects.
2. To observe that increased heart rate and blood pressure recorded during a particular calisthenic will change from student to student while the oxygen requirement for that activity remains constant.
3. To understand the importance of monitoring the cardiovascular changes that occur during a low intensity exercise.

STEP 1: EXPERIMENTAL PROCEDURES

1. Divide class into two groups, A and B. Group A will perform exercise A and group B will perform exercise B. The remaining instructions are the same for both groups.

Exercise A

Count 1 bilaterally abduct shoulders to horizontal "T" position
Count 2 flex elbows, bringing hands toward shoulders
Count 3 extend elbows, returning to "T" position
Count 4 return to anatomical position

Exercise B: Sitting with Legs Hanging Off the Edge of Plinth

Count 1   extend right knee
Count 2   flex right knee
Count 3   extend left knee
Count 4   flex left knee

2. For each student performing the exercise, one student is needed to record heart rate (palpate) and one student is needed to record blood pressure (sphygmomanometer). See the Appendix at the end of Exercise 9 for instructions on how to take heart rate and blood pressure measurements.

3. There are four variations of each exercise. The student should perform each variation of the exercise in random order. Steps 4 and 5 are to be followed during each exercise bout.

   Slow continuous—perform the exercise at 60 counts per minute

   Slow pause—perform the exercise at 60 counts per minute; exercise during counts 1–4, then pause on counts 5 and 6; begin exercise with count 1.

   Fast continuous—perform exercise at 120 counts per minute.

   Fast pause—perform exercise at 120 counts per minute; exercise during counts 1–4; pause on counts 5, 6, 7 and 8; begin exercise on count 1.

4. Set timer for 4 minutes. Set the metronome. Allow the student to practice the exercise. Begin when student is ready.

5. During the last 30 seconds of minute 4, measure blood pressure. Obtain heart rate value during the last 10 seconds of minute 4. Record values on Table 10-1. Calculate rate pressure products ($HR \times SBP$).

6. Complete Figures 10-1, 10-2, and 10-3 with bar graphs representing heart rate (1), systolic blood pressure (2), and the rate pressure products (3) during each variation of the exercise.

Discussion Questions

1. Compare the rate pressure products obtained from the four methods of performing the calisthenic. Did your results coincide with the studies performed by Greer and DiCarlo?[3]

2. Compare your results (Figures 10-1, 10-2, and 10-3) with those of other students. Were you able to see different cardiovascular responses among students in your class for the same exercise?

Table 10-1 Cardiovascular response to 4-minute exercises.

Variation	Heart rate (beat/min)	Blood pressure (mmHg)	Rate pressure ($HR \times SBP$)
Slow continuous			
Slow pause			
Fast continuous			
Fast pause			

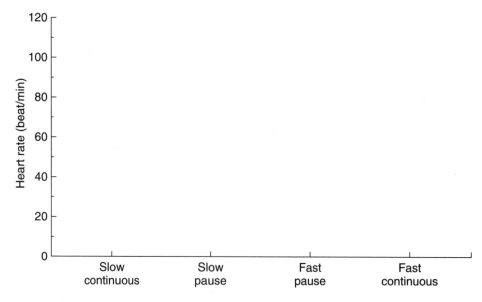

Figure 10-1 Heart rate response to four variations of the exercise.

3. Were the hemodynamic responses of students who performed exercise A different from those who performed exercise B?

4. Discuss the limitations of using METS to prescribe exercise. Refer to the previous exercise, Laboratory Exercise 9, Step 3, Case Study 1. Would any activities prescribed for the gentleman be dangerous for him to perform, even though the MET value for the activity is within the safe range?

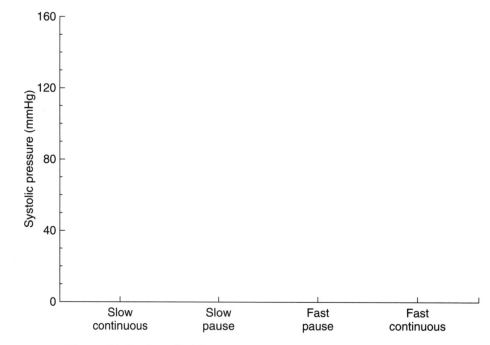

Figure 10-2 Systolic blood pressure response to four variations of the exercise.

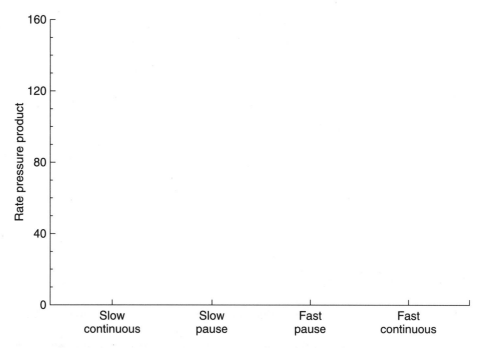

Figure 10-3   Rate pressure product response to four variations of the exercise.

NOTES

1. Greer et al., "Heart Rate and Blood Pressure Response," 179–83.
2. DiCarlo and Leonardo, "Hemodynamic and Energy Cost Responses," 1585–90.
3. Greer, "Physiological Responses," 1146–51; DiCarlo and Leonardo, "Hemodynamic and Energy Cost Responses," 1585–90.

LABORATORY EXERCISE 11: CALCULATION OF THE MOMENT OF FORCE

BACKGROUND AND THEORY

The following exercise will involve determining the moment of force of muscle contraction during isometric, isotonic, and isokinetic exercise. The muscle moment of force or torque developed during muscle contraction will be recorded during each type of contraction. You will be able to observe any change in moment of force that results from changing the joint angle and the differences in moment of force produced by three different types of contractions.

Skeletal muscle is composed of numerous muscle fibers. The sarcolemma covers the muscle fibers, fuses with the tendons, and inserts into the bone. The muscle fibers consist of several hundred to several thousand myofibrils. Within each myofibril, there lies approximately 1500 myosin filaments and 3000 actin filaments. The actin and myosin filaments, also referred to as thin and thick filaments, respectively, are large protein molecules responsible for muscle contraction. Electron micrograph of myofibrils will appear banded because of the interdigitation of the actin and the myosin filaments, Figure 11-1.

The light bands or I-bands are regions which only contain the actin filaments. The dark bands or A-bands contain myosin filaments and regions where actin and myosin overlap. The ends of the thin filaments join at the Z-disc and extend in both directions, interdigitating with myosin filaments. The region between consecutive Z-discs is a **sarcomere**. The length of the sarcomere is approximately 2 microns when the muscle fiber is elongated to its resting length.

The sliding filament theory may help to account for muscle contraction (Figure 11-2), in which the actin filaments slide across the myosin filaments via cross bridge linking. Cross bridges are extensions of the myosin filament which can bind to the myosin binding sites on the actin filaments. Neither the actin filaments nor the myosin filaments change in size during contraction. In the **contractile state** of the fully shortened muscle, the actin filaments are maximally overlapping each other and the Z-lines have been pulled up to the end of the myosin filaments (part D, Figure 11-2). The muscle can be stretched to the extent that the actin filaments are too far from each other and there are no cross bridges linking actin and myosin filaments (part A, Figure 11-2). In either state (part A or part D), the tension developed by muscle contraction is minimal. The sarcomere can generate its greatest force of contraction at the point where actin filaments completely overlap the myosin filaments, maximizing cross bridge formation (Figure 11-2, part C). The

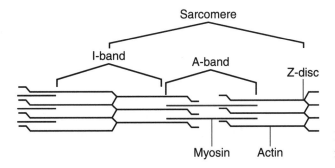

Figure 11-1   Actin and myosin filaments of the myofibril.

events involved in muscle contraction have been described in Exercise 7 if you need to review excitation-contraction coupling.

Contraction of the entire muscle under the influence of length variations is the summated effect of contractions of its individual fibers. The whole muscle follows the same laws that govern a single muscle fiber. Therefore, there exists an optimal muscle length (L_{max}) at which the maximum tension is produced.

In addition to the length-tension relationship illustrated in Figure 11-3, a relationship exists between the load being lifted by the muscle and the speed of contraction (Figure 11-4). As the load on the muscle increases, the rate of contraction decreases. Notice on Figure 11-4 that the force generated at zero velocity corresponds to the maximum isometric tension. We will demonstrate the force-velocity relationship using the isokinetic dynamometer.

When considering the force required to lift/displace a given load, one should also consider the mechanical relationship of the body's anatomical **lever system,** in which the angle of muscle pull and the length components of the lever system are involved in moving a load. This is an important consideration because the torque of a muscle varies as a result of different angles of pull throughout the limbs' range of motion, and there exists an angle at which the muscle is performing (generating force) maximally.

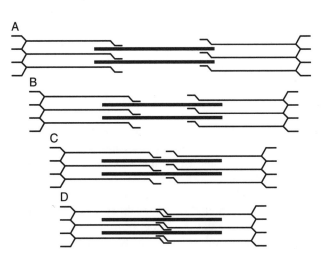

Figure 11-2   Sliding filament theory in which the actin filaments slide across the myosin filaments. In part A, the actin filaments are far apart. The tension developed under these conditions is small. The actin filaments are closer together in part B. This allows more cross bridges to form between the actin and myosin filaments and more tension can be developed as a result. There is more overlap of actin and myosin filaments in part C, maximizing the cross bridge formation and the tension generated in the muscle fiber. Further overlap of actin and myosin filaments is shown in part D. Notice that the actin filaments overlap each other as well. Under this condition, the muscle fiber cannot generate any more tension. Refer to the length-tension relationship illustrated in Figure 11-3. The letters on the graph correspond to the letters in this figure.

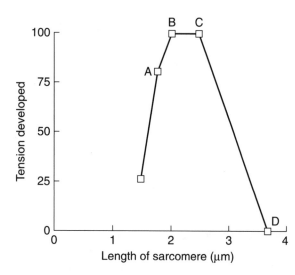

Figure 11-3   The length-tension diagram indicates that there exists an optimal sarcomere length at which the greatest tension is produced. Notice that the optimal length is not when the sarcomere is at its greatest length. The optimal length corresponds to the length of the sarcomere when the actin filaments completely overlap the myosin filaments for maximum cross bridge attachment.

To better understand the concept of a muscle's ability to generate force, let us look at a simple equation which specifies that a condition for equilibrium has been established,

$$M \times MA = R \times RA$$

$$M = \text{moment}$$

$$R = \text{resistance}$$

$$MA = \text{moment arm}$$

$$RA = \text{resistance arm}$$

where M is the moment of force or torque required to move the weight, MA is the perpendicular distance from the line of action of muscle force to the axis of rotation (joint), R is the weight to be lifted, and RA is the perpendicular distance from the joint to the weight (R). MA, RA, and R are easily obtained; therefore the moment of force (M) required to lift or move the load through the range of motion can be calculated. It is important to note that force and torque are not equivalent. Torque is a force applied over a lever arm that causes rotation. It is also important to note that the equation above states a condition of equilibrium, i.e., there is no rotation.

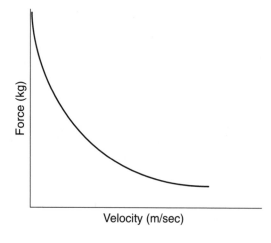

Figure 11-4   The force-velocity relationship states that as the speed of a concentric muscle contraction increases, the maximum force generated by the muscle decreases. This can be demonstrated by counting the number of times you can lift a five pound weight in thirty seconds and compare that with the number of times you can lift a fifteen pound weight in thirty seconds.

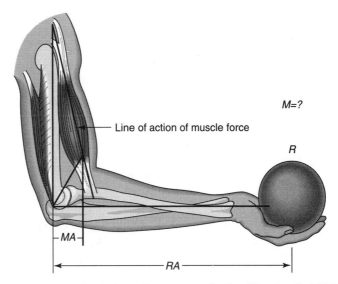

Figure 11-5 Calculation of torque required to lift a load of 10 kg at a 90° angle.

$R = 10$ kg, $RA = 10$ cm, $MA = 2$ cm, $M = \underline{\quad}$ kg, $M \times MA = R \times RA$, $M \times 2 = 10 \times 10$, $M = 100/2$, $M = 50$ kg.

However, the moment of force shifts the curve to the left and torque or movement occurs. To illustrate this concept, a sample calculation was performed in Figure 11-5.

Suppose the angle was changed such that *the elbow was flexed. R* is the only parameter that remains the same (Figure 11-6).

The force required to lift the weight is less and will be perceived by the individual as "lighter" even though *R* is the same in both examples. The equation and

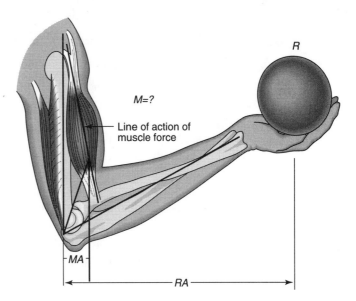

Figure 11-6 Calculation of torque required to lift a 10 kg load at a 45° angle.

$R = 10$ kg, $RA = 8$ cm, $MA = 1.7$ cm, $M = \underline{\quad}$ kg, $M \times MA = R \times RA$, $M \times 1.7 = 10 \times 8$, $M = 80/1.7$, $M = 47$ kg.

graph incorporate the mechanical advantage of the length of the lever arms (moment and resistance arms) and the angle of pull.

> *How would* M *change if the* MA *increased?*
>
> *How would* M *change if the* RA *increased?*

The muscle force may be considered a resultant force that can be decomposed into two constituent forces: rotary and joint compressive. The size of each component depends upon the angle at which the force is applied. If the force is perpendicular to the segment being moved, the segment moves in a rotating direction. If the force is parallel to the segment being moved, the segment moves in a parallel or compressive direction. The basic idea is this: as joint angles increase up until the point where the muscle-tendon complex is pulling at 90 degrees to its bony lever, there will be a constant change in the proportion or ratio of compressive to rotary forces. That is, the rotary force progressively increases, thus affording more torque (turning force) about the joint axis while (joint) compressive forces decrease, decreasing the joints' inertia and tendency to remain stationary. This explains clinically why subjects/patients have difficulty initiating movements. However, once movement starts, further motion becomes easier. The reverse scenario is therefore also true. As the angle of insertion gets smaller, the compressive forces increase while the rotary forces decrease. There are two extremes here, one practical and one theoretical. If the muscle-tendon is at 90 degrees to the lever, then there is only rotary force (i.e., no compression exists). The other case is theoretical. If the tendons' line of pull could become parallel with its lever (it cannot since this would mean that the tendon would have to fall inside the boundary of the neutral axis of the bone), then the force would be all compressive with no rotation.

There are both physiological and mechanical advantages involved in muscle contraction and maximum tension generated. The **length-tension** concept states that the maximum tension generated by the muscle occurs at its resting length when there is the greatest number of cross bridges between myosin and actin. However, there are optimal angles at which the maximum moment of force or torque can be generated throughout a joint range of motion. The idea of locating the point at which the maximum muscle moment of force can be generated is relevant to exercise training and rehabilitation to increase muscle strength according to the overload principle.

There are three different methods of resistance training used to increase muscle strength. **Isometric** exercise involves muscle contraction without muscle shortening; it allows maximum loading, but only at one point in the range of joint motion. Isometric contractions can, however, be performed at various joint angles to accomplish resistance training throughout the joint range of motion. During conventional **isotonic** exercise, the external resistance or weight remains the same throughout the range of motion, i.e., free weights. Due to the anatomical lever system, the moment of force or torque of the muscle are not constant throughout the range of motion; the load selected can only be as great as what can be moved at the weakest point in the range of motion and therefore the rest of the system will work at less than capacity. Moving through the joint's range of motion consists of a shortening or **concentric** contraction and a lengthening or **eccentric** contraction. Maximal loading at each point in the joint range of motion is possible with **isokinetic** exercise. The exercise is performed at a controlled speed such that the effort applied encounters an equal counteracting moment of force. Maximal contraction is possible at each point in the range of motion because increasing the muscle movement only increases the resistance or resisting movement, not the rate of movement.

An isokinetic dynamometer is a measuring device which can be set at various speeds to offer resistance at every point in the range of motion proportional to the force exerted; the device generates a record of the torque exerted by the muscle group. Torque is the product of the rotational force applied over a lever/movement arm distance which is the perpendicular distance between the joint axis and the line of pull of the muscle. Maximal force generated during eccentric contraction is greater than the force produced during isometric contraction. The force generated during isometric contraction is greater than that produced during concentric contraction.

ECCENTRIC > ISOMETRIC > CONCENTRIC

You will compare the torque output of the knee extensors, knee flexors, elbow extensors, and elbow flexors during isometric, isotonic, and isokinetic contraction.

Materials

isokinetic dynamometer, dumbbells (free weights)
goniometers or electrogoniometer

Student Objectives

1. To differentiate between isometric, isotonic, and isokinetic resistance exercise.
2. To understand the length-tension diagram and be able to differentiate between the physiological and biomechanical limitations of torque output.
3. To observe changes in torque associated with muscle contraction at different joint angles.
4. To be familiar with the an isokinetic dynamometer in assessing muscle strength.

STEP 1:   EXPERIMENTAL PROCEDURES

This experiment was designed for the student to compare the torque output of the knee/elbow extensor and flexor muscles during isometric, isotonic, and isokinetic contractions.

Divide the class into two groups, A and B. One or more members of Group A will demonstrate isometric, isotonic, and isokinetic contractions with knee flexion/extension. One or more members in Group B will perform the exercises with elbow flexion/extension.

Knee Flexion/Extension

Isokinetic, isometric, isotonic
1. Subject should sit on the testing table, leaning on the backrest.
2. Stabilize the subject at the shoulders, waist, and distal portion of the thigh. Attach the testing device 4 cm above the medial malleoli of the dominant leg.

3. The limb should be aligned with the lever arm of the dynamometer. Align the anatomical axis of rotation of the knee joint with the rotational axis of the dynamometer.

4. Set the dynamometer to 30°/second. Subject should perform a few practice repetitions, complete knee flexion and extension.

5. To complete the isokinetic exercise, the subject should perform three maximum flexion-extension cycles.

6. Allow subject to rest one minute between each cycle.

7. Set the dynamometer to 180°/second; complete the isokinetic exercise as in the previous steps.

8. To perform the **isometric** exercise, set the dynamometer to 0°/second.

9. The subject should perform one maximal contraction at every 10 degrees in the range of motion (90° to 20° or 10°).

10. **Isotonic** contractions will be performed using the one repetition maximum procedure. Your instructor will instruct you on the procedure for determining one repetition maximum for concentric and eccentric contractions. The one repetition maximum consists of the maximal load that can be lifted once.

Elbow Flexion/Extension

Isometric, isotonic, and isokinetic
1. Subject should lie on the testing table (supine with hips and knees flexed).
2. Stabilize the subject at the shoulders and legs. Attach the testing device to the forearm of the subject, just proximal to the wrist.
3. Supinate the forearm; the forearm should be aligned with the lever arm of the dynamometer. Align the axis of the elbow joint with the rotational axis of the dynamometer.
4. Set the dynamometer to 30°/second. Subject should perform a few practice repetitions, complete flexion and extension.
5. To complete the isokinetic exercise, the subject should perform three maximum flexion-extension cycles.
6. Allow subject to rest one minute between each cycle.
7. Set the dynamometer to 180°/second; complete the isokinetic exercise as in the previous steps.
8. To perform the **isometric** exercise, set the dynamometer to 0°/second.
9. The subject should perform one maximal contraction at 30°, 45°, 60°, 90°, 110°, 130°, and 150°.
10. **Isotonic** contractions will be performed using the one repetition maximum procedure.

Discussion Questions

1. From the dynamometer printout, trace a torque-joint angle curve for knee or elbow extension at both speeds on Figure 11-7 or 11-8. Plot the torque produced from isometric muscle contraction at specific angles on the same graph. One isometric and two isokinetic torque-joint angle curves should be on the same graph.

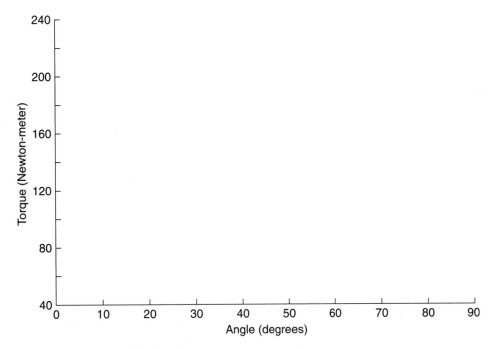

Figure 11-7   Torque-joint angle curve for knee extension.

2. From the dynamometer printout, trace a torque-joint angle curve for knee or elbow flexion at both speeds on Figure 11-9 or 11-10. Plot the torque produced from isometric muscle contraction at specific angles on the same graph.

3. Within the isometric contraction exercises, at which angle was the greatest muscle moment of force produced? During an isometric contraction the muscle is not shortening. Biomechanically, suggest an explanation as to why this joint angle produced the greatest moment of force.

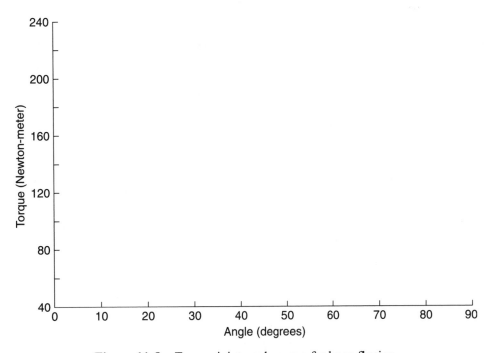

Figure 11-8   Torque-joint angle curve for knee flexion.

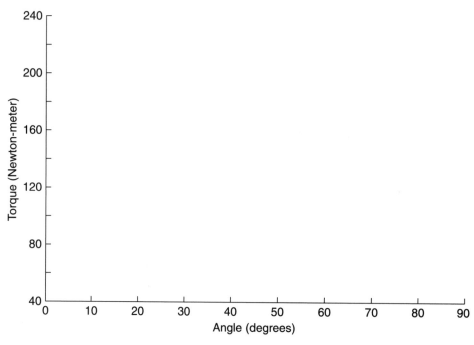

Figure 11-9 Torque-joint angle curve for elbow extension. Plot points for isometric and isokinetic contraction.

4. Interpret the results of the isokinetic exercise. At which angle was the greatest moment of force produced according to the range of motion/torque curve obtained from the dynamometer?

5. Compare the one repetition maximums for the concentric and eccentric portions of the contraction. It has been documented that the moment of force

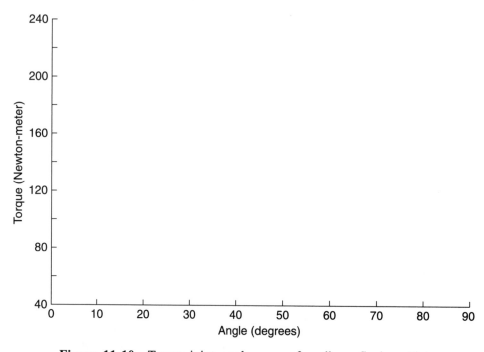

Figure 11-10 Torque-joint angle curve for elbow flexion. Plot points for isometric and isokinetic contracton.

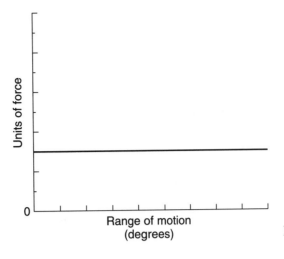

Figure 11-11

output is greater during eccentric contraction, i.e., elbow extension involves lengthening of the biceps brachii and knee flexion involves lengthening of the quadriceps femoris. It is important to note that concentric and eccentric moment of force during a task are not the same as maximal eccentric and concentric moment of force capability. This is why, for any task, you are closer to your concentric moment of force maximum than your eccentric moment of force maximum. How do your results compare?

6. Which method of resistance exercise produced the greatest muscle moment of force (torque output)?

7. During conventional isotonic exercise, the external resistance or weight remains the same throughout the range of motion and can be illustrated in the Figure 11-11. The straight line represents the external force at the skeletal lever, i.e., the external force is constant.

   Complete the graph (Figure 11-12) representing the percentage of muscle moment of force capacity used throughout the range of motion. Would you expect the percent muscle moment of force capacity to be the same throughout the entire motion?

8. During the isokinetic exercise, the resistance moment at the skeletal lever changes. The resistance is variable and accommodates the ability of the subject.

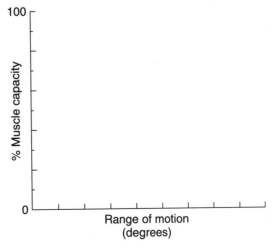

Figure 11-12

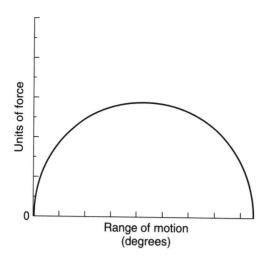

Figure 11-13

The hyperbola represents the force at the skeletal lever, i.e., the moment of force changes during isokinetic contractions (Figure 11-13).

Complete the Figure 11-14 representing the percentage of muscle moment of force capacity used throughout the range of motion during isokinetic contractions.

9. The isokinetic exercise was performed at two speeds, 30°/second and 180°/second. Which speed produced the greatest torque output? Previous studies have demonstrated that as the concentric velocity increases, the muscle torque output decreases. Is this the case?

➡️ *Point of Interest*

The limitations of muscle contraction can be physiological or biomechanical. Two or more joint muscles sometimes exhibit **passive insufficiency.** To demonstrate this concept, sit on the floor with knees extended and dorsiflex the ankle; notice that the gastrocnemius is fully stretched, limiting further dorsiflexion. Now flex the knee a little and dorsiflex the ankle again. The amount of dorsiflexion should be greater because the gastrocnemius is slack (not fully stretched) and does not limit the action

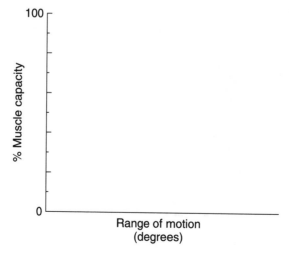

Figure 11-14

of dorsiflexion. You can use a string to represent the gastrocnemius; place the string on the surface of the gastrocnemius during knee extension and pull it taut. When the knee is flexed, the string should be slack.

Physiologically, a muscle can only shorten to approximately 50% of its resting length. We confront this limitation when we make a simple fist. If we flex the wrist before we try to make a fist, our grip strength is reduced. The flexor digitorum superficialis muscle involved in flexion of the wrist is also involved in flexion of the fingers. Once the flexor digitorum superficialis contracts during wrist flexion, a fist cannot be formed in that hand because the muscle cannot shorten to the degree required to flex the fingers and form a fist. This concept is referred to as **active insufficiency.** A tight fist also *cannot* occur because the long finger extensions cannot lengthen enough (passive insufficiency). The instructor and students may also choose to make a fist with slight wrist hyperextension versus wrist flexion. Please observe and record your observations.

Most muscles have a **primary** and a **secondary action.** For example, the primary function of the biceps brachii muscle is elbow flexion; its secondary action is supination of the forearm. The elbow and forearm muscles involved in using a screwdriver (if you are right handed and turning the screw clockwise) are the supinator, brachioradialis, and biceps brachii muscles. You may have experienced the difficulty of keeping the head of the screwdriver in the groove of a screw. The screwdriver may actually jerk out of the groove as a result of the primary action of the biceps brachii (elbow flexion) overriding its secondary action (supination). The triceps brachii prevents the strong elbow flexion action of the biceps brachii so that the biceps brachii can strongly supinate.

LABORATORY EXERCISE 12: AN ELECTROMYOGRAPHIC ANALYSIS OF ISOMETRIC, ISOTONIC, AND ISOKINETIC CONTRACTIONS

BACKGROUND AND THEORY

Laboratory Exercise 11 provided an introduction to muscle contraction and the moment of force generated by the active muscle during isometric, isotonic, and isokinetic contraction. We will build on that exercise by observing the electrical activity elicited by the three different types of contractions using electromyographic techniques. It may be helpful to review the events of excitation-contraction coupling described in Exercise 7. The functional unit of muscle contraction is the motor unit, consisting of the motor neuron and the muscle fibers it innervates. Motor neurons extend from the anterior horn of the gray matter of the spinal cord, branch and innervate the individual muscle fibers. The location of nerve innervation of the muscle is the motor point. The number of motor neurons and the firing frequency of impulses from the motor neurons determine the force of muscle contraction.

The rate of action potential initiation at the sarcolemma (motor end plate) is a determinant of skeletal muscle performance. The more rapid the rate of action potential initiation, the stronger the muscle contraction because muscle contractions will summate with time (temporally). The force of a temporally summed contraction is greater than the force of a single contraction. The increase in muscle force developed as a result of multiple action potentials firing in rapid succession is referred to as temporal summation. Contractions may sum to the extent in which they will fuse and appear as a single, sustained contraction, called *tetany* (Figure 12-1).

Electromyography (EMG) is a powerful technique for studying muscle function; it can also be used to study the relationship between EMG output and muscle force. Surface electrodes are sufficient for measuring activity in superficial musculature from which gross representation of activity is desired. It is important to note that muscles deep to the superficial muscles may also be monitored by the same electrode. The signal obtained from surface electrodes, however, may be attenuated due to large amounts of subcutaneous fat. Fine wire electrodes may be inserted into the muscle to study specific motor units; however, only surface electrodes are required for this laboratory exercise. The largest signals are obtained when the recording electrode is placed over the motor point, i.e., the location in which the nerve innervates the muscle. Once a motor point of the muscle has been identified, it should be used to obtain consistent results.

Due to individual differences in subcutaneous fat and muscle geometry, between subject comparisons involve normalizing the data. Clinicians and

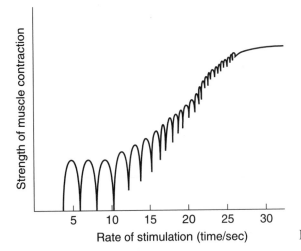

Strength of muscle contraction

Rate of stimulation (time/sec)

Figure 12-1   Temporal summation.

researchers often translate the values from a test or procedure to a percentage of the EMG produced during a maximal voluntary contraction. The EMG produced during a maximal contraction is obtained prior to the test or procedure. In this way, the EMG recording is normalized as a percent of the individual's maximum.

The type of muscle contraction, changes in muscle length during the contraction, and the various methods of gathering EMG data have prevented the precise EMG-tension relationship from being defined. It was established years ago that muscle length altered the relationship of EMG to muscle tension such that EMG decreased while muscle tension increased beyond resting length.[1] The investigators observed the greatest electrical activity in the triceps when the muscle contracted to its shortest length, a length associated with the lowest moment of force (torque). The decreased electrical activity recorded with increasing muscle length may be due to the presence of less muscle mass beneath the electrode to generate the EMG. Also, at longer muscle lengths, the nervous system perceives the muscle to have more tension. Consequently, the Golgi tendon organ senses an increased tension and inhibits the alpha motor neurons, which diminishes the resulting EMG, Figure 12-2.

It is also important to note that there is an increased muscle-tendon unit moment of force when the muscle is elongated beyond its resting length due to the summation of contractile elements as well as passive connective elements.

This laboratory exercise will employ the EMG technique to examine the difference in electrical activity among isometric, concentric, eccentric, and isokinetic contractions. Previous studies have demonstrated that there is a linear relationship between EMG and muscular force during isometric contractions in large muscle groups, i.e., muscles of the limbs, while smaller muscle groups produce a curvilinear relationship between EMG and force. Later researchers found that concentric contractions (muscle shortening) elicited greater electrical activity than eccentric contractions (muscle lengthening) when the velocity of shortening and lengthening was held constant.[2] Conversely, the maximal muscle torque output during concentric contractions is less than the maximal muscle torque output during an eccentric contraction. Dynamic contractions are difficult to evaluate due to muscle length changes during the contraction and the time course of the contraction.

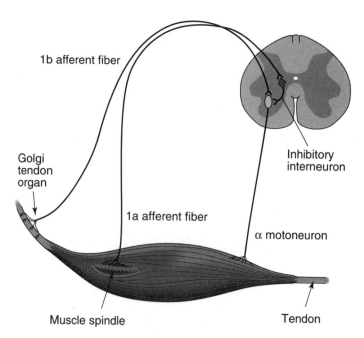

Figure 12-2   The Golgi tendon organ (GTO) responds to a change in tension or force, unlike the muscle spindle which responds to a change in length. In response to an increase in tension, the Golgi tendon organ sends signals to the spinal cord via the 1b afferent fiber. The 1b fiber synapses with an inhibitory interneuron. The interneuron synapses with the alpha motoneuron and has an inhibitory effect.

Materials

electromyograph recording device
goniometer
dynamometer, free weights

Student Objectives

1. To compare the electrical activity of the muscle elicited by isometric, concentric, eccentric, and isokinetic contractions.
2. To compare EMG and muscle torque output for each type of contraction.
3. To be familiar with EMG recording.

STEP 1:   EXPERIMENTAL PROCEDURE

1. Divide the class into two groups, A and B; forming the same groups as in the previous lab may be helpful in analyzing the results. Performing the procedure on the same volunteers is not necessary but would be to your advantage in comparing the EMG data with the muscle torque output.
2. Palpate the rectus femoris/biceps brachii to locate the center of the muscle. Clean the skin with alcohol, apply conductive paste to the area and place the

surface electrode at this point. The second electrode should be placed a short distance away parallel to the muscle fibers. To eliminate any stray electrical activity, place the ground electrode at a point where there is minimal muscle between the skin and the bone.

3. The student should assume the proper position for isometric contraction on the isokinetic dynamometer, as performed in Laboratory Exercise 11. Complete the same procedure.

4. The same procedure as in Laboratory Exercise 11 will also be used for the isokinetic and isotonic contractions.

5. Plot the EMG activity for isokinetic and isometric contractions on Figures 12-3 and 12-4 for elbow flexion and extension, or on Figures 12-5 and 12-6 for knee flexion and extension.

6. Compare the angles at which the maximum tension was produced in Laboratory Exercise 11 with the angles at which the greatest EMG activity occurred.

7. EMG is determined/calculated by normalizing the responses to the EMG activity evoked during a maximal voluntary contraction (MVC). Subjects/students are asked to perform a MVC and the maximum EMG activity is recorded. All subsequent responses are normalized as a percent of the maximum EMG.

Elbow flexion isotonic; **IEMG activity:**

Elbow extension isotonic; **IEMG activity:**

Knee flexion isotonic; **% of max IEMG activity:**

Knee extension isotonic; **% of max IEMG activity:**

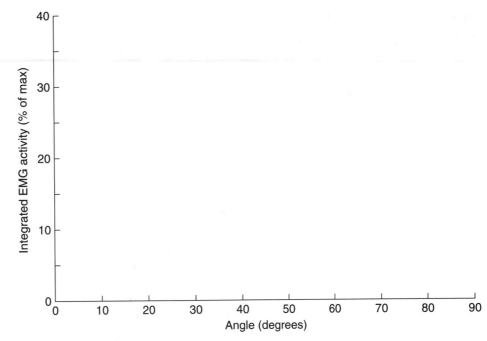

Figure 12-3   EMG activity during isometric and isokinetic contractions at various angles of elbow flexion.

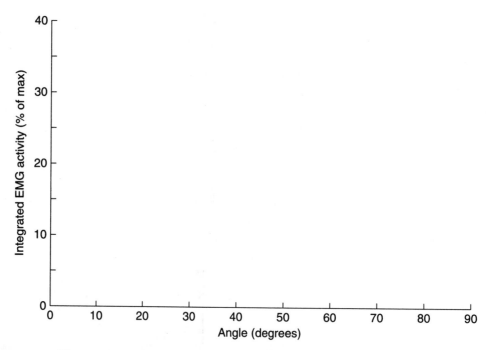

Figure 12-4   EMG activity during isometric and isokinetic contractions at various angles of elbow extension.

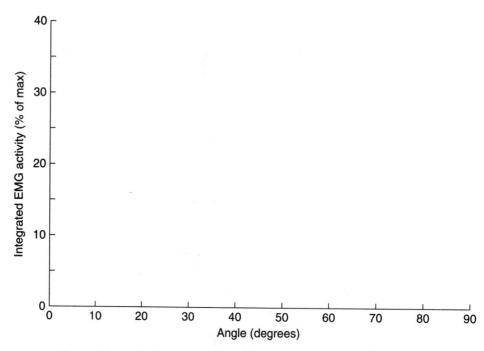

Figure 12-5   EMG activity during isometric and isokinetic contractions at various angles of knee flexion.

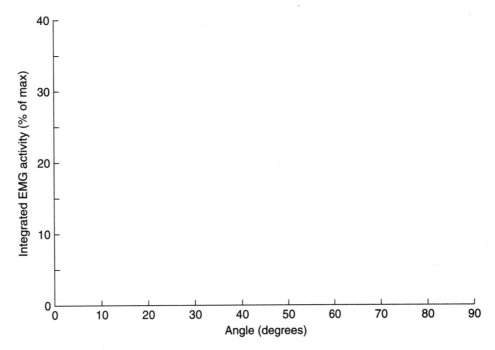

Figure 12-6   EMG activity during isometric and isokinetic contractions at various angles of knee extension.

Discussion Questions

1. Which type of contraction produced the greatest IEMG activity? How does this compare with the type of contraction which generated the greatest muscle moment of force?

2. At which angle (isometric or isokinetic contraction) was the electrical activity of the muscle greatest? How does this correspond to the angle which produced the greatest muscle moment of force?

3. If the electrical activity recorded in the muscle did not change significantly, with increased tension developed, what other factor is important in determining muscle moment of force?

4. It has been shown that there is greater electrical activity during concentric muscle shortening than eccentric muscle lengthening for the same task. How do your results compare?

NOTES

1. Inman et al., "Relation of Human Electromyogram to Muscular Tension," 187–94.

2. Bigland and Lippold, "The Relation between Force, Velocity, and Integrated Electrical Activity," 214–24.

Select Bibliography

INTRODUCTION

Basmajian, J. V. "Professional Survival: The Research Role in Physical Therapy." *Physical Therapy,* 57(3):283–285, 1977.

Basmajian, J. V. "Research of Retrench: The Rehabilitation Professions Challenged." *Physical Therapy,* 55(6):607–610, 1975.

Hislop, H. J. "The Not-So-Impossible Dream." *Physical Therapy,* 55: 1069–1080, 1975.

Johnson, D. W., R. Johnson, and K. A. Smith. *Active Learning: Cooperation in the College Classroom.* Edina, MN: Interaction Book Co., 1991.

Michels, E. "Physical Therapy Research: The Crucial Challenge for the Future." *Progress Report of the American Physical Therapy Association,* 17: 6, 1988.

Reynolds, J. P. "Towards the 21st Century in PT Education." *PT Magazine,* November: 54–62, 117–118, 1993.

Schon, D. *Educating the Reflective Practitioner.* San Francisco: Jossey-Bass, 3–21, 1987.

EDUCATIONAL APPROACH

Matyas, M. L. "Teaching by Inquiry: What Is It? Why Do It?" *The Physiologist,* 41(1): 43, 1998.

Vander, A. J. "The Excitement and Challenge of Teaching Physiology: Shaping Ourselves and the Future," *American Journal of Physiology,* Advances in Physiology Education, 12(1): 53–516, 1994.

LABORATORY EXERCISE 1

Portney, L. G. *Planning Clinical Research,* 128–132, 1980.

Zar, J. H. *Biostatistical Analysis (2nd edition).* Englewood Cliffs, NJ: Prentice Hall, Inc. 307–310, 1984.

LABORATORY EXERCISE 2

Nelson, R. and G. Hunt. "Strength-Duration Curve: Intrarater and Interrater Reliability," *Physical Therapy,* 61(6):894–897, 1981.

Portney, L. G. *Planning Clinical Research,* 33–34, 1980.

Riddle, D. L., J. M. Rothstein, and R. L. Lamb. "Goniometric Reliability in a Clinical Setting." *Physical Therapy,* 67(5):668–672, 1987.

Zar, J. H. *Biostatistical Analysis.* Englewood Cliffs, NJ: Prentice Hall, Inc., 1984.

LABORATORY EXERCISE 3

Golding, L., C. Myers, and W. E. Sinning, Eds. *Y's Way to Physical Fitness: The Complete Guide to Fitness Testing and Instruction,* 3rd edition. Human Kinetics Publishers, 108–110, 1989.

Moritani, T. and H. A. DeVries. "Neural Factors Versus Hypertrophy in the Time Course of Muscle Strength Gain," *American Journal of Physical Medicine,* 58(3):115–130, 1979.

Portney, L. G. *Planning Clinical Research,* 38, 56–57, 1980.

DeLorme, T. L. and A. L. Watkins. "Techniques of Progressive Resistance Exercise." *Arch. Phys. Med.* 29: 263–273, 1948.

LABORATORY EXERCISE 4

Griffin, J. E. and T. C. Karselis. *Physical Agents for Physical Therapists.* Springfield, IL: Charles C. Thomas, 8, 14, 148–152, 161–164, 1980.

Shriber, W. J. *A Manual of Electrotherapy.* Philadelphia: Lea & Febiger, 23, 28–34, 1975.

LABORATORY EXERCISE 5

Gibbon, J. H. and E. M. Landis. "Vasodilation in Lower Extremity in Response to Immersion of the Forearm In Warm Water" *Journal of Clinical Investigation,* 11(9):1019–1036, 1932.

Griffin, J. E. and T. C. Karselis. *Physical Agents for Physical Therapists.* Springfield, IL: Charles C. Thomas, 153–159, 1980.

Kerstake, D. M. and K. E. Cooper. "Vasodilation in the Forearm in Response to Heating the Trunk, *Journal of Physiology,* 110(12):24, 1949.

Lehmann, J. F. and B. J. DeLateur. "Therapeutic Heat." In *Therapeutic Heat and Cold.* J. F. Lehmann, Ed. Baltimore: Williams & Wilkins, 430–431, 444–445, 1984.

Jackins, S. and A. Jamieson. "Use of Heat and Cold in Physical Therapy." In *Therapeutic Heat and Cold.* J. F. Lehmann, Ed. Baltimore: Williams & Wilkins, 646–656, 1984.

Taylor, W. F. and V. S. Bishop. "A Role for Nitric Oxide in Active Thermoregulatory Vasodilation." *Am. J. of Physiol.* 264(Heart & Circ. Physiol. 33):H1356–1359, 1993.

Stillwell, K. G. "Therapeutic Heat." *Physical Medicine and Rehabilitation.* 233–243, post 1960.

LABORATORY EXERCISE 6

Griffin, J. E. and T. C. Karselis. *Physical Agents for Physical Therapists.* Springfield, IL.: Charles C. Thomas, 13–17, 1982

Lehmann, J. L. and B. J. DeLateur. "Cryotherapy." In *Therapeutic Heat and Cold.* J. L. Lehmann, Ed. Baltimore: Williams & Wilkins, 1990.

Olson, J. E. and V. D. Stravino. "A Review of Cryotherapy." *Physical Therapy.* 52(8): 840–853, 1972.

Urbscheit, N. and B. Bishop. "Effects of Cooling on the Ankle Jerk and H-Response." *Physical Therapy.* 50(7):1041–1049, 1970.

LABORATORY EXERCISE 7

Griffin, J. E. and T. C. Karselis. *Physical Agents for Physical Therapists.* Springfield, IL.: Charles C. Thomas, 13–17, 1982.

Shriber, W. J. *A Manual of Electrotherapy.* Philadelphia: Lea & Febiger, 23, 28–34, 1975.

LABORATORY EXERCISE 8

Guyton, A. C. *Textbook of Medical Physiology.* Philadelphia: W. B. Saunders Company, 184, 281, 369; 1991.

LABORATORY EXERCISE 9

DiCarlo, S. E. "Effects of Aerobic Fitness in Hemodynamic Responses to Upright Tilting." *Physical Therapy.* 68(8):1204–1208, 1988.

DiCarlo, S. E. and P. I. Wolfe. "Fatigue Rate During Anaerobic and Aerobic Exercise in Insulin-Dependent Diabetics and Nondiabetics." *Physical Therapy.* 63(4):500–504, 1983.

Sinning, W. E. *Experiments and Demonstrations in Exercise Physiology.* Philadelphia: W. B. Saunders Co., 55–59, 1975.

LABORATORY EXERCISE 10

Greer, M., S. Dimick, and S. Burns. "Heart Rate and Blood Pressure Response to Several Methods of Strength Training." *Physical Therapy.* 64(2):179–183, 1984.

Greer, M., T. Weber, S. Dimick, and R. Ratliff. "Physiological Responses to Low-Intensity Cardiac Rehabilitation Exercises." *Physical Therapy.* 60(9):1146–1151, 1980.

DiCarlo, S. and J. Leonardo. "Hemodynamic and Energy Cost Responses to Changes in Arm Exercise Technique." *Physical Therapy.* 63(10):1585–1590, 1983.

LABORATORY EXERCISE 11

Falkel, J. "Plantar Flexor Strength Testing Using the Cybex Isokinetic Dynamometer." *Physical Therapy.* 58 (7):847–850, 1978.

Gaslin, B. R. and J. Charteris. "Isokinetic Dynamometry: Normative Data for Clinical Use in Lower Extremity (Knee) Cases." *Scandinavian Journal of Rehabilitative Medicine.* 11: 105–109, 1979.

Guyton, A. C. *Textbook of Medical Physiology.* Philadelphia: W. B. Saunders Company, 1991.

Hislop, H. and J. Perrine. "The Isokinetic Concept of Exercise." *Physical Therapy.* 47(2): 114–117, 1967.

Knapik, J. J. "Isometric, Isotonic, and Isokinetic Torque Variation in Four Muscle Groups Through a Range of Joint Motion." *Physical Therapy.* 63(6):938–947, 1983.

Luttgen, K. and K. Wells. *Kinesiology: Scientific Basis of Human Motion.* Philadelphia: CBS College Publishing, 1982.

Murray, M. P., G. M. Gardner, L. A. Mollinger, and S. B. Sepic. "Strength of Isometric and Isokinetic Contractions: Knee Muscles of Men Aged 20 to 86." *Physical Therapy.* 60(4):412–419, 1980.

Scudder, G. N. "Torque Curves Produced at the Knee During Isometric and Isokinetic Exercise." *Archives of Physical Medicine & Rehabilitation.* 61(2):68–73, 1980.

Thompson, C. W. *Manual of Structural Kinesiology.* Boston: Times Mirror/Mosby College Publishing, 1989.

LABORATORY EXERCISE 12

Bigland, B. and C. J. Lippold. "The Relation between Force, Velocity, and Integrated Electrical Activity in Human Muscles." *Journal of Physiology (London).* 123:214–224, 1954.

Inman, V. T., H. J. Ralston, and C. M. Sanders. "Relation of Human Electromyogram to Muscular Tension." *Electroencephalography Clinical Neurophysiology.* 4:187–194, 1952.

Komi, P. V. "Relationship Between Muscle Tension, EMG and Velocity of Contraction Under Concentric and Eccentric Work." In Desmedt, J. E., Ed.: *New Developments in Electromyography and Clinical Neurophysiology,* vol. 1. Basel, Switzerland: Karger, 596–606, 1973.

Soderberg, G. L. and Cook, T. M. "Electromyography in Biomechanics." *Physical Therapy.* 64(12):1813–1820, 1984.

Rosentswieg, J. and M. Hinson. "Comparison of Isometric, Isotonic and Isokinetic Exercises by Electromyography." *Archives of Physical Medicine & Rehabilitation.* 249–260, 1972.

Guyton, A. C. *Textbook of Medical Physiology.* Philadelphia: W. B. Saunders Co., 1991.

Olson, J. E. and V. D. Stravino. "A Review of Cryotherapy." *Physical Therapy.* 52(8): 840–852, 1972.